Recovering the Nation's Body

Recovering the Nation's Body

*Cultural Memory,
Medicine, and the
Politics of Redemption*

Linda F. Hogle

Rutgers University Press

New Brunswick, New Jersey, and London

Library of Congress Cataloging-in-Publication Data

Hogle, Linda, 1953–
     Recovering the nation's body : cultural memory, medicine, and the
politics of redemption / Linda F. Hogle.
          p. cm.
     Includes bibliographical references and index.
     ISBN 0–8135–2644–2 (cloth : alk. paper). — ISBN 0–8135–2645–0
(pbk. : alk. paper)
          1. Allocation of organs, tissues, etc.—Germany—Public opinion.
     2. Public opinion—Germany.   3. Allocation of organs, tissues, etc.—
     United States—Public opinion.   4. Public opinion—United States.
     5. Transplantation of organs, tissues, etc.—Social aspects—
     Germany.   6. Transplantation of organs, tissues, etc.—Social
     aspects—United States.   7. Transplantation of organs, tissues,
     etc.—Moral and ethical aspects—Germany.   8. Transplantation of
     organs, tissues, etc.—Moral and ethical aspects—United States.
     I. Title
     RD126.H64   1999
     362.1'783'0943—dc21
                                                                           98–45601
                                                                           CIP

British Cataloging-in-Publication data for this book is available from the British
Library

Manufactured in the United States of America

Dead material should be for us nothing more than the illustration of life. . . . The goal of the living should be to understand and assess it.
—Rudolf Virchow, quotation placed
at the entry to the Virchow Anatomical
and Pathological Exhibit, Berlin

Every cell, every tissue is a part of us that doesn't belong in someone else's body.
—opposer of organ donation,
field notes, March 1994

Contents

Figures and Tables

Figures

Tables

Acknowledgments

My ideas for this interdisciplinary work developed from varied sources. I owe much to the pioneers of science and technology studies, bioethics, and anthropology, who by preparing the field have enabled a growing number of mingled projects to flourish.

Without key sources of support, for which I am deeply grateful, the project would not have been possible. My research in Germany was funded by a Fulbright Fellowship, and secondary and follow-up research was funded by the University of California President's Fellowship, the Chancellor's Graduate Research Fellowship, a Graduate Research Award, and two PEO Scholar Awards.

I wish to thank many people for their participation and help, primarily the transplant coordinators and surgeons, managers, activists and opponents, politicians, theologians, and others who generously shared their thoughts about difficult and sensitive issues. I am grateful to Bernward Joerges for inviting me to be a guest scholar at the Wissenschaftzentrum für Sozialforschung, Berlin. I was also invited as a guest in the Science History and Theory Section of the Förderungsgesellschaft Wissenschaftliche Neuvorhaben Berlin, which allowed me additional time for follow-up and refinement. Sabine Helmers, Ingo Braun, Karin Knorr-Cetina, Ingelore and Beate Gumlich, Trevor Pinch, Patty Marshall, Judith Barker, and Monica Casper were wonderful sources of intellectual exchange and, on occasion, of practical aid and rescue. In particular, I thank Volker Schmidt for his help-ful and lively exchanges. His discipline as a scholar inspired me, and I ap-preciate the good humor with which he handled my attempts to understand German society. Also enriching my experience in Germany were Annedore Schulze and Wilfried Pommerahnke, who taught me the true meaning of German hospitality and how to share life's joys and difficulties.

I am fortunate to have had several readers who combined critical acuity with stimulation and encouragement. Early on, I benefited from the wisdom of Margaret Clark, Paul Rabinow, and Barbara Koenig. Thanks also to David Hess, Uli Linke, Deborah Heath, Sarah Franklin, and Dorothy Nelkin for reading early drafts. Joe Dumit made thorough and thoughtful comments, as did Adele Clarke—a mentor, friend, solace, and constant support. Finally, just as any work consists of more than theories and artifacts, this book ex-ists because of the enthusiasm and expertise of my editor, Martha Heller, and the patience and perseverance of my research assistant, Molly Harrod.

Recovering the Nation's Body

One

Introduction

Situating Medical Practices

In an old German folktale, a wolf approaches a herd of sheep.

"Do you know me?" says the wolf.

"I know your type," says a sheep.

The wolf explains that he is not a danger but a friend to sheep because he eats only dead sheep that are left to rot in the field. "I don't eat live sheep. Couldn't I just stay by the herd in case one of you dies?" he asks.

The sheep forbids him, saying, "An animal that eats dead sheep learns quickly out of hunger to see sick sheep as dead ones and then healthy ones as sick ones."

This story, reproduced in old German script, is the frontispiece to one of the many books published in Germany during the early 1990s about organ transplantation and brain death (Hoff and in der Schmitten 1994). The authors intend the tale to serve as a warning about German medicine, which they claim waits for any opportunity to use the bodies of the flock for its own purposes. The story captures the feelings of mistrust and fear common in postwar Germany as well as outside its borders and addresses utilitarian justifications for the use of bodily materials from the vulnerable to benefit others in society. Similar images have been used by other critics, including journalists, physicians, politicians, and theologians, who draw a more direct comparison to the abuses of medical and state authorities under National Socialism. They warn that allowing powerful medical or

1

governmental authorities to prey upon the powerless, such as the brain dead, can too easily expand to include all members of society.

The use of biological materials from the human body—organs, tissues, and cells—evokes intense and diverse reactions. Acquired primarily from bodies that are still physiologically functioning but have been declared brain dead, these materials are used for organ and tissue replacement, research, and pharmaceutical preparations. Does harvesting tissue violate bodily integrity? Does it show disrespect for the dead or dying? Does it use technology for unnatural purposes or function as an abuse of control over a powerless flock? Or is it the "ideal use of our remains," as one physician put it, an efficient recycling of waste material, a reasonable use of a valuable resource? Is it an altruistic gesture, sharing life-giving matter with those who need it?

This book is about the removal and use of human bodily materials in contemporary Germany. I pay particular attention to the way in which various meanings of the body affect and are affected by cultural, medical-technical, and legal practices. Such interactions unfold in unique ways in different settings, even within Euro-American environments that are often presumed to be homogenous. That is, they can change according to the relation of the state and other authorities to individuals in society and through the addition of new technologies or modified views of old ones. They can also change through attempts to overlay religious, economic, and political frames. The interplay between old and new, secular and sacred, technical and cultural has profound implications in terms of who societies allow to make decisions about the rights and protections of bodies, what constitutes violation of or rightful access to useful resources, and how these resources are defined and valued for legal, regulatory, and commercial purposes.

Medical practices related to these extraordinary materials are carried out in different ways within particular contexts, social arrangements, and organizational structures. "Universal" medicine is viewed through the lens of national and transnational politics, economics, and history. How, then, does one account for differences among geographically bounded areas or within ethnic, religious, or other groups?

To explore these various questions, I conducted ethnographic research in Germany, where the historical, social, and political contexts surrounding the use of humans and human materials are unique. Contemporary practices of collecting and using parts of human bodies are played out against the history of medicine under National Socialism, in which living and dead bodies were used for a variety of experimental and commercial purposes. Humans were a cheap and accessible source for tissue culture; bodily materials from freshly killed prisoners were used for study, while skin and bones were recycled into other products and sold. Thus, any use of materials from some humans for the benefit of others recalls the Nazis' large-scale social-medical projects meant to extend the capabilities and prospects of select humans at the expense of others. Furthermore, as in Japan and some other countries, the issue of redefining death has raised the specter of abuse. This fear is particularly acute in Germany: its history of euthanizing "lives not worthy of living" resurrects the question of who has the right to proclaim which bodies are dead, how those bodies will be used, and who will benefit.

There are other histories as well. Centuries-old concepts of continued animation in dead bodies, codified in law and evident in cultural practices, reverberate through contemporary debates over defining brain death. For example, the ways in which bodies in Germanic territories were handled at death and the use of cadaver materials for healing purposes sheds light on past and present understandings of the body at death. More recently, the relationship between the East German socialist state and its citizens suggested that bodies were virtually state property. The Stasi's secretive collections of bodily fluids, odors, and other materials used for citizen identification and the state's use of the dead for medical purposes without permission makes contemporary Germans very suspicious about the intervention of state or medical authorities into the private bodies of citizens.

Studying the Body as a Therapeutic Tool

The body is an object of renewed interest in the social sciences. Yet theories of the body's relationship to self and society are polarized between an unproblematized view of biology without context and a view that reduces the body to little more than language and representation.

Without losing sight of important discursive formulations of the body, I chose to place the materiality of the body in the foreground. By centering on human materials as healing agents, I was able to study the various participants involved and the relations among them. I also focused on the *procurement* processes of materials—that is, the removal and processing procedures that transform raw human body parts into implements for therapy or research. In this way, I was able to follow the interactions between everyday activities and political and social movements, economic trends, institutions, and organizations. My approach differs from existing studies of transplantation and other end uses of tissue, which consider either the experiences of living patients who receive these therapies or policies concerning the tissue's allocation. My study, then, does not reexamine arguments about the propriety of using parts of some human bodies to forestall the death of others. Nor does it study personhood per se or offer an abstract theory about the fragmentation of bodies in modernity. Rather, I examine the body as a source of and site for therapeutic tools and consider bodily constituents as instruments and technological artifacts that are both culture bearing and profit bearing.

The Body, Technology, and Society

We live in an age in which people expect technology to create solutions for physical limitations. Organ transplantation has become one such way to replace failing body parts and forestall death. But why use human bodily materials rather than develop other alternatives to therapy? One answer is that synthetic materials and devices have mechanical and biocompatibility problems, are expensive and time-consuming to develop, and involve complex arrangements between research and manufacturing organizations, funding sources and regulatory agencies. Moreover, the complicated physiology of organs such as livers cannot easily be duplicated.

It took years to develop tissue substitution into a workable therapy. In addition to medical expertise, it required infrastructure, policies, financial reimbursements, and other arrangements—all of which involved both private corporations and the state. In Foucault's terms, science and the state's concern for the vitality and productivity of bodies was linked to these instrumental means for gaining control.

Recently, there has been a tremendous increase in demand for whole organs and tissues, not only because of the many patients who may die without them but also partly because medical research has devised many new applications for them. For example, organ replacement used to be reserved for end-stage organ failure. Now, however, it is also considered an option (although a controversial one) for genetic abnormalities, cancer, and meta-bolic disorders. New uses and improved techniques require many types of tissue and organs: pancreas, intestines, lungs, ear bones, dura mater, um-bilical cord stem cells, and endothelial cells, to name a few. Cells, tissues, and organs go into diagnostic reagents and are used in research and com-mercial applications (cf. Koebe and Shildberg 1994).

The image of a perpetual shortfall of supply in the face of growing de-mand is central to rhetoric about organ and tissue donation. Hence, fictional films and books, folktales (such as the one about the wolf), and urban myths reflect a general concern about aggressive attempts to acquire materials. Anthropologist Nancy Scheper-Hughes (1996) has provided insight into such images from popular culture as well as lay views and perceptions about organ donation, particularly among vulnerable populations.

Social scientists are studying organ substitution as a complex and chal-lenging medical technology, and there has been a resurgence of interest in theorizing the body. In their classic article, Nancy Scheper-Hughes and Margaret Lock (1987) call into question basic concepts determining how the body is perceived in both biomedicine and anthropology. Beginning from the view of the body as "simultaneously a physical and symbolic artifact, both naturally and culturally produced," they warn against reproducing (or uncritically taking on) biological assumptions characteristic of western bio-medicine. This movement of interest in the body has spawned a diversity of literature that uses the body to rethink social relations.[1] Bryan Turner, in particular, has problematized taken-for-granted categories of biological and cultural aspects of humans (1987, 1992). While acknowledging the ex-istence of real pain and biological sources of disease and disorder, these works use the body as a model in more symbolic and metaphoric ways.

The relation between technology and the human body has received grow-ing attention since the 1980s.[2] Still, in general such considerations do not focus on scientific and biomedical practices and the ways in which knowl-edge about the body is produced by various actors in these domains. Fur-ther, when these writers study the effects of technology *upon* society or the body, they often presume that science, technology, and medicine operate in a sphere entirely different from society.

Work from the interdisciplinary area known as science and technology studies is changing this deterministic view, suggesting that transformations are more interactive between a variety of actors and occur in a variety of settings.[3] Recent works have explored not only the blurring of bodily boundaries but who is involved in the process. Other perspectives examine how bodily transformations parallel processes in the global economy in the late twentieth century by moving through a number of settings where such transformations occur.[4]

Cultural studies writers have suggested that, in view of evolving communications and medical technologies, the body is being transformed or is disappearing altogether under conditions of late capitalism.[5] While earlier works used machine metaphors and production analogies to describe processes, these new works make explicit the fact that boundaries between bodies and technologies have already been crossed. As Marilyn Strathern (1992: 60) has said, "the concept of culture is already problematised. It is not at all clear what is or is not an artefact. The point is not that the boundaries between bodies and machines are theoretically troublesome, but that we now live in a world that makes explicit to itself the ability to breach the difference." Strathern has captured the idea that the anthropological concept of culture has been based upon the secure knowledge that we know what is natural and can thus understand what—and how—things become cultural. The destabilization of that knowledge is central to being able to analyze late twentieth-century uses of the body.

Crossing the border of the natural and the cultural challenges cultural classifications that attempt to maintain the separation between the domains of material objects and persons. Complicating these distinctions is the fact that often materials are removed from bodies that are physiologically functioning with the aid of technology but are legally and medically defined as dead—brain dead. The categories of live and dead, human and nonhuman, natural and technological have been imploded, with profound implications for how these ambiguous entities are defined, how their use is organized and controlled, by whom, and for what purposes.

Such constructions of meaning are consequential. The ways in which the body is conceptualized influence ways in which health care is planned and delivered. The increasing array of implants and artificial devices challenges concepts of self, alters the patient-physician relationship, and brings manufacturers, regulators and state authorities, lawyers, and insurers more directly into that relationship.

Materials from human bodies have multiple cultural, political, and symbolic meanings, but in their use as therapeutic and research tools they are material objects as well. They are perishable, organic objects with economic value that must be managed through cultural mechanisms. Human biological materials thus have characteristics and properties that pose particular opportunities and constraints.

There are few good models for studying human materials themselves in their role as research and therapeutic tools. In contrast, studies of specific uses of the body—organ transplantation, in particular—have focused on a range of issues related to either identity transformation or policy. These include studies of personhood and the body as it relates to the recipient of the materials (Sharp 1995) and philosophical or legal perspectives regarding treatment of the body, the body as property, or health services aspects dealing with costs, quality of life, and meanings for organ recipients (Joralemon 1995, Mathieu 1990).[6] Renée Fox and Judith Swazey's influential works have been the cornerstone of social science perspectives on organ substitution. *The Courage to Fail* (1974) has helped practitioners, ethicists, and social scientists think through the issues and implications. But in *Spare Parts* (1992), they change their position from hopeful if cautious optimism to deep concern, as the commercialization and aggression with which the technologies are pursued is becoming more apparent.

Related issues concern the legal and social constructions of brain death and the ethics of using the brain dead as donors (Lock and Honde 1990, Ohnuki-Tierney 1994). Margaret Lock's groundbreaking work in Japan (1995, 1996) provides comparative data that contribute not only to our understanding of changing conceptions of death but, more important, challenge the way in which social scientists—North Americans in particular—have perceived other societies' responses to technologies as exotic.

My research both supports and departs from these perspectives, showing how the valuation, usefulness, and meaning of human materials comes not simply from abstract theorizing but from the material practices of negotiating definitions and classifications, arranging exchange systems, and managing the technical constraints of procurement and distribution of human materials. This approach requires going to the core of scientific and technological practices, including an examination of the elaborate if often invisible infrastructures that must be in place for any procurement to occur.

In the words of Clarke and Fujimura (1992: 3), "medical work is enabled or constrained by the accessibility, cost and pacing associated with specific tools for scientific jobs. . . . Doing science involves multiple different tools, processes, and participants and their articulation across time and space."

This perspective is nuanced by the growing body of literature that examines scientific practice—that is, what scientists actually do—rather than focusing solely on structures, interests, or particular individuals or institutions (Hacking 1992, Pickering 1992). These routine, everyday practices are integral to changes in the way in which the body and its materials are conceptualized, including the shifting of borders between persons and things. To be usable as therapeutic tools or exchangeable as commodities, human body parts must undergo a series of conversions. These processes are best demonstrated by works on nonhuman creatures—for example, Clause (1993), Kohler (1994), and Lynch (1988), which demonstrate specific processes through which organisms are altered and commodified, including certain ritual aspects around the organism that help researchers separate the domain of thing (research tool) from living being.

The work of classifying human materials as usable material for therapy or other purposes, as sacred remains, or as anything else inherently involves a system for valuing. Kopytoff (1986), among others, notes that such classifications and assigned values of objects are not static. Rather, their status as commodities or as items outside the realm of exchangeable objects changes under different conditions and over time.

Moreover, value changes according to the intended purpose. For example, in the case of human materials to be used for therapy, especially in organ transplantation, the viability of the organ—its ability to animate—increases its value. But simultaneously the body of the person from whom it was removed must take on a different status. This is where practices become most contested. Human materials and their sources have politics; that is, there are programs and agendas built into them that regulate authority relations and access to the means of production.

Germany, Medicine, and the Global Economy

Much attention has been devoted to globalizing processes in the late twentieth century. Some social scientists see the outcomes as homogenizing. Indeed, there have been intense efforts in a number of industries, including medicine, to standardize protocols and procedures, to create a universalized medicine. Observing a combination of effects, however, several anthropologists have challenged this idea, finding that globalizing forces have created a great deal of diversity. Their work points to the significant role that imagining and forgetting plays in the reconstruction of identities and communities.[7]

If we apply these important contributions to the study of scientific communities, it becomes clear that people have made distinctions between western and nonwestern medicine, and even distinctions within western medicine, that they assume to be unproblematic. As Gupta and Ferguson (1992: 14) explain, "there is a unity of 'us' and an otherness of the 'other.'" Social studies of science and technology have in large part concentrated on western industrialized nations but in doing so have often ignored the connections to nonwestern societies and discontinuities between cultures that are assumed to be similar. Even though many people explicitly recognize the effects of time and space compression in production and information flows, the weakness in their arguments has been their failure to recognize the creolization and hybridization of knowledge production as it occurs within locales.

A few researchers have contemplated the nature of differences between organizational and academic structures across nations.[8] Given the sullied past of national character studies, however, this is precarious business among anthropologists (Neiberg and Goldman 1998). Looking for distinctions is extremely difficult in the case of Germany. Just mentioning the country's name conjures all sorts of images in the minds of many people. It is difficult to tease apart stereotypes—outsiders' imagination of their community—in the politics of representation (Forsythe 1989).

Germany within the European Union

What might constitute difference within the politically constructed borders of the nation is also confounded by the political aesthetics of connection to the European Union (EU). Participation in the global economy is a central concern in Germany. Medical technologies and practices are not separate from policies and activities in this regard. To participate in transnational exchange of scientific, technological, and medical knowledge as well as financial profits, German institutions must use similar procedures, have equivalent facilities, and have infrastructures that articulate with those of international research partners to enable work to proceed (Vollmer 1994).

A move toward standardization is a central feature of Germany's participation in the EU. Imposing standardized rules based on universal principles is meant to enable the transnational flow of capital and goods—critical in the late twentieth-century global economy. More than simply an economic trading bloc, the EU is a matrix of political, social, and economic ministries to which member countries are expected to cede much of their authority. Local working and living conditions are affected as these supranational institutions set policy for finance, manufacturing, trade, and even social welfare programs across all member countries. As the experience of several industrial and welfare segments has shown, this can engender considerable resistance and form complicated logistical barriers.

To facilitate transnational trade within Europe, policymakers in the 1980s and early 1990s made intense efforts to harmonize all policies and standards, including health and safety codes, pricing policies and subsidies, production and quality indices, and even hiring requirements. But if it is a formidable task to make centuries-old, family-owned breweries conform to large-scale industrial manufacturing standards for the beverage industry, then it is a Herculean task to harmonize medical and ethical practices across national regulatory structures, medical and political jurisdictions, and legal systems, not to mention cultural and religious beliefs. What, then, about tissue removed from the dead, which in some countries is legally classified as a human biological, in others as a medical device or pharmaceutical? Since World War II, German laws and guidelines regarding research on and use of human materials have been among the strictest in the world.[9] Nevertheless, various EU commissions are attempting to standardize classifications, pricing, and regulations, and the Council of Europe (1994) has written several sets of recommendations for ethical guidelines for medical practice.

In addition to establishing political and financial links among member nations, the EU has attempted—quite unsuccessfully—to develop a supranational cultural identity among the peoples of Europe. In a way, this acknowledges that identities in late capitalism are formed in ways not tied to geographic boundaries.[10] There are, after all, informal and formal links between communities of practice in most enterprises. Certainly this is true in medicine, where physicians identify with others in their specialty despite national boundaries. They establish scientific, educational, and commercial connections with colleagues and attempt to create common languages of practice to facilitate the movement of goods, people, theories, and techniques across borders. Such links have been crucial to the successful development and expansion of human materials use.

Ironically, while the physicians I spoke to during my research insisted that it was possible and necessary to standardize the science of transplant medicine across nations (medicine as acultural and universal), they often placed their subjects in explicitly cultural frames. For example, one respondent was perplexed about the German population's unwillingness to embrace organ donation, comparing the situation to a "similar" cultural group: "In Austria they have an autopsy law and a [presumed consent] transplant law, and they have no problem with it. They cannot be so far away from us: culturally, spiritually, ethically, and morally we are similar. So why is there such a problem here?" (surgeon, f.n., September 1994).

Communities of practice transect expected boundaries and build on other notions of identity: competence, similarity, belonging. In turn, identities, whether national, professional, or local, figure into policy and decision making at all levels. When I asked questions about Europe-wide practices and techniques in organ procurement, I often encountered physicians' stereotypes of others: "You can't put Holland and Belgium in the same group with the GDR—you defame them [the Dutch and the Belgians]" (West German surgeon discussing the surgical techniques of East Germans, f.n., September 1994).

Within the EU, Germany occupies an awkward yet important position. Europe both needs and fears a strong Germany. Yet at the time of this writing, Germany, which has been one of the strongest supporters of a united Europe, did not meet the financial criteria for continued membership. With about 11 percent unemployment (up to 25 percent in parts of the eastern region) and debt greater than 3 percent of the gross domestic product, the prospects are not exactly sunny (Fritsch-Bournazel 1992). Germany is thus being pressured externally by its European neighbors and internally by a myriad of new social and economic difficulties. The addition of tens of thousands of immigrants seeking asylum and the extraordinary expense of reunification have also created great financial strain.

Medical science and technologies, which have been industrial mainstays in Germany, are seen as a way to stimulate industry and employment for the future (Schicke 1988). Transplant medicine is an answer to many chronic, expensive illnesses and a highly profitable and growing industry as well. An aging population and increasing public interest in better therapies to justify higher medical costs is stimulating this demand for life-extending technologies. In short, there is a technological and economic imperative to expand the once-premier biomedical industry, which has fallen behind in global competition.

East Meets West

After World War II, Germany was split by an artificial physical border, and two distinct political, economic, and ideological cultures emerged.[11] The reunification of Germany has created new problems in the reconstruction of German identity. According to the mayor of Leipzig, "No one . . . had any idea how far apart we had grown in 40 years. I can tell you if West Germany had absorbed Italy or France, the problems would have been far less than they are with the absorption of East Germany" (quoted in the *New York Times,* October 14, 1994, p. A1).

John Borneman (1992a, b) eloquently describes the implications of this division on identity, noting that on both sides of the border elements of pre-twentieth–century German history were combined with particular state images of the "ideal" German set against "other" Germans:[12]

> [Germans'] relation to *die drüben,* those over there . . . , was based on pure fantasy. For the West Germans, the connection rested on a projection of the meaning of Germanness onto the other: *Ossies* were a mirror-image, a replica waiting to join them in a whole Germany. For the East Germans, fantasies of the West were formed primarily by images from West German television: *Wessies* are the desired other, richer, more successful, more powerful. (Borneman 1992b: 24)

These images have dissolved into distinct stereotypes:

> "The Ossies are like caged animals; they don't know what to do when they are set free." (f.n., June 1994)

> "Ossies are like apes from the zoo; after being captured for so long, they can't survive on their own without being told what to do." (f.n., June 1994)

"Wessies are all so narcissistic and arrogant. They just spend money on themselves and don't care about anything. They adopted this from America." (f.n., September 1995)

"Wessies think they're so much better than us—we've had the same training, we're intelligent too, but they don't look at our abilities, just where we're from." (f.n., July 1994)

Millions of Deutschmarks are being spent on the physical reconstruction and administrative reorganization of all public services in the east to dismantle Communist structures and "catch the East up to West German standards," as respondents often reminded me. Entire infrastructures are being rebuilt: phone systems, roads, railways, postal codes, banking, and monetary systems are still in the process of complete overhaul.

These same processes are paralleled in medicine.[13] In the former East Germany (the GDR), medical care was centralized in Berlin, with major centers in the larger cities. This meant that outlying areas lacked facilities for both acute and chronic care, such as dialysis clinics. Services focused on prevention and primary care, while sophisticated technology was concentrated only in the major centers, primarily Berlin. As they have done with the rest of the economy, Western "experts" have moved in to modernize and increase the number of facilities, replacing the politically organized administration with western-style management.[14]

A plethora of new opportunities for profit-based medicine has come with the colonization of eastern medical systems. The number of new dialysis centers in the east has doubled since 1990 (H. Schmidt 1994). Western physicians call this growth "catching up in quality and quantity of care," but the other side of the story is that private clinics represent a profitable growth industry and an attractive opportunity for entrepreneurial physicians who are struggling with the glut of hospital-based physicians in the west. A large number of eastern physicians were fired after being accused of complicity with the Stasi, leaving high-level university posts vacant.[15] More often than not, these positions were filled by western physicians, who were offered huge incentives to move to the "less desirable" east. Higher status, plentiful government research funding to "develop" the east, cheap lab space, and less stringent regulations have attracted a number of clinicians, researchers, and investors (*Frankfurter Allgemeine Zeitung* 1994a).[16] The skilled, less expensive workers in the former GDR are not only more available but are perceived as being more docile and compliant than the "spoiled" workers in the west. Like the rest of the work force, medical personnel in the east—including physicians—are employed in lower-level positions and make 20 to 30 percent less in salary than their western counterparts, even those employed by the same organizations.

These differences have caused a culture clash of management and organizational styles, methods, and types of interaction with patients and staff. In eastern hospitals I visited, staff and physicians resented the arrogance of westerners, who treated them like ignorant, inexperienced dolts. They resisted western administration policies mandating that patients should be refused treatment if the insurance fund will not pay. They missed the feeling of solidarity: in their words, working together as a team and having less social distance between job roles. In West German clinics, staff resented the lack of autonomy (often described as laziness) and lack of skills among East German nurses. In general, West Germans believed that East German staff at all levels were unwilling to work beyond what was minimally required and that administrative policies in the former GDR were hopelessly inefficient because they had been tied to party politics.

Stereotypes and rumors on both sides were pervasive. To elicit their decision-making patterns in various situations, I occasionally asked physicians to respond to hypothetical scenarios.[17] No matter what the example, western physicians often responded with something like "oh, that could only happen in the east," then giving explanations that usually mentioned the more compliant nature of eastern nurses or the general incompetence of eastern hospital staff and physicians. Responding to the identical scenario, eastern physicians responded with "that must have happened in the west because . . . ," giving explanations that concerned the arrogance of western physicians or the lack of cooperation or solidarity among workers. Both sets of physicians then explained how they would proceed in the west or the east. Not only did they respond first to the eastern or western components of the situation rather than to the nature of the scenario itself; their interpretations of what had happened and how the situation would be dealt with was colored by their idea of who they themselves were. In short, stereotypes from other parts of society are reproduced in medical practice, influencing work and relationships. Mistrust on both sides means that physicians often blame each other if the quality of tissue is poor or if the way in which it was procured is not perceived as proper.[18]

Clearly, a particular combination of political, economic, historical, and cultural contexts shapes medical practices that concern the use of bodily materials. In the wake of global and regional changes and continued controversy over the role and authority of medicine, it is not surprising that the number of materials voluntarily made available for use in Germany has decreased significantly. This contrasts with other countries, where organ and tissue donation is rising.[19] The appendix shows these changes in donation rates as well as listing responses to surveys about attitudes and willingness to donate—revealing some interesting differences between Germans in the former eastern and western states.

Procuring Information

My intent in this multisite ethnography was to show the multiple contexts and thus the broader cultural meanings within which the various interpretations of human materials technologies make sense.[20] Medicine, after all, is practiced not only at the bedside and in the operating room but at the telephone and the computer, in the offices of governing bodies, in community meetings, and at social gatherings. At each of these sites, medical work cannot be separated from social activities and meanings, and participants move through many different social worlds.

Central to my argument is the idea that transformations take place where local, everyday practices interact with global economic, social, and political contexts. As Arjun Appadurai (1986: 5) suggests, the meanings of things are "inscribed in their forms, their uses and their trajectories. . . . it is the things-in-motion that illuminate their human and social context." Thus, I examined how materials are circulated across regional and national borders and organizational boundaries. Although I could not travel with a liver to its ultimate destination in another country, I followed its virtual path through information and tracking systems. I also attended transnational meetings where exchange policies and problems were debated among transplant professionals.

Primarily, though, I observed the procurers. Following what these participants actually do—their mundane and everyday activities—illuminated local-global intersections just as clearly as they showed how hands-on practices reflect local understandings of the body at death. I observed all routine activities of the coordinators and surgeons most intimately associated with procuring materials. Their activities included data handling, coordination of logistics for potential donors, clinical management of brain-dead donors, removal of materials in the operating room, and follow-up work.[21] I observed these procedures in hospitals and university clinics in cities throughout all parts of Germany. My most intensive observations took place in Berlin, where reunification has created a unique and problematic merger of facilities, personnel, and techniques undergirded by political and territorial disputes. The research was conducted over a sixteen-month period in 1993 and 1994, with a follow-up visit in 1995. Previously, I had conducted a seven-month ethnographic study of an organ procurement organization in the United States, which provided invaluable information on bedside practices, institutional issues, and exchange mechanisms.

I interviewed physician and nonphysician coordinators, medical researchers collecting and using the materials, transplant surgeons who used organs, pathologists, nursing staff in operating rooms and intensive care units, and others such as social workers and pastoral staff who work in clinical settings. I included managers and administrators of procurement and exchange organizations in Germany and at the transnational organization in the Netherlands. While formal interviews yielded information about reactions to public resistance and personal interpretations of legal, cultural, and medical-scientific aspects of organ procurement, my observations allowed me to locate points of conflict and commitment and to consider how these points mediate between cultural meanings and the technical aspects of procurement.

I found many other rich sources of information about how Germans perceive organ procurement: theologians, political activists, journalists, and representatives of groups opposed to the use of human materials. At various stages I interviewed politicians and lawyers involved in regulating the procurement and allocation of human tissue. During the course of my research, I attended a number of public "town hall" discussions about organ donation and brain death—a marvelous opportunity to observe the direct interactions (often hostile) among concerned individuals, transplant surgeons, and city or regional government officials. Informal conversations with friends and colleagues not directly involved in procurement practices or debates were also a useful source of information, particularly when they discussed their reactions to media coverage and their own beliefs and traditions regarding the body at death and the appropriate use of human bodies.

This book is not a comparative study; I focus on Germany historically and within its own set of contexts. Nevertheless, readers unfamiliar with the technologies and practices involved may find it helpful to have another case for comparison. For this reason, I occasionally introduce examples from my ethnographic research in the United States, where I observed an organ procurement organization in a single metropolitan area. These examples are intended to illustrate the local and contingent nature of practices, not to make the United States the case against which other situations should be evaluated.

Harvesting Information from This Book

The book is broken into two parts: part 1 surveys the historical, cultural, and legal fields in which bodily materials are used; part 2 focuses on the actual practices of procurement in Germany, including the infrastructural elements that make the enterprise possible.

Part 1

Part 1 discusses the cultural meanings of the body at different times in German history. Chapter 2 considers how the body is handled at death, including funerary customs as well as various medical, commercial, and other uses for body parts. Chapter 3 concentrates on the unique history of the body during National Socialism. Chapters 4 and 5 move to contemporary issues. The development of legal notions of body integrity—and when these notions may shift—is discussed in chapter 4, along with political implications. Chapter 5 demonstrates how recent public spectacles showing particular uses of human bodies have revealed layers of old conceptions while encouraging newer ways of thinking about the relationships among the body, technology, and the state.

The information in part 1 ranges over a broad area for two reasons: to create a backdrop for part 2 and to provide a glimpse of the complex environment in which organ and tissue recovery proceeds in Germany. Medical practices are deeply rooted in German and European history and geography and must also be considered within a global economic frame.

Part 2

Clearly, the work of transforming human tissue into therapeutic tools consists of scientific and technical aspects that cannot be separated from social and political aspects. In part 2 I show these connections by examining the infrastructural elements that must be in place for the technologies to exist and suggesting how local practices both formulate and are affected by these structures. Readers who are particularly interested in transnational trade and policy issues may want to concentrate on chapters 6 and 7. In chapters 8 and 9 readers will find information about the procedures themselves, including the hands-on aspects of removing organs and tissues. I end the book in chapter 10 with some thoughts about ways in which the use of human bodily materials reflects broader social concerns in Germany. As such, it demonstrates ways that German society, including medicine, struggles to reformulate itself at the end of the twentieth century.

A combination of foresight and pure luck brought me to Germany at the peak of the controversy over the use of human materials and the struggle to find legal and moral answers. I quickly learned that the social conflicts of reunification, its economic and competitive pressures, and the process of coming to terms with the past were no backdrop to the scene; they were central to the story. Some of the most technical medical issues are rooted in Hanseatic or Prussian ways of doing business, and colonialist attitudes toward East Germans are linked to knowledge about what and whose organs will work. The interconnections are extraordinarily complex, resulting in a book that some might call too broad-ranging. Nevertheless, this complexity is precisely what I want to portray.

My intention is neither to vilify nor to venerate practices of procuring and using human materials. The people I spoke to had strong opinions and often had expectations of the work. They wanted to know which side I was on, and undoubtedly some readers will ask the same question. My purpose, however, is simply to show what is involved in converting human biological materials into usable therapeutic tools in the particular conditions of late twentieth-century Germany.

Part I

German Culture, History, and Boundaries of the Body

S tudying the procurement and use of human biological materials (HBM) as therapeutic and research tools is a unique opportunity to examine medical sciences and technologies under the political and economic conditions of the late twentieth century. But there are a number of alternative sources of knowledge about the body, each of which has something to say about the relation of the organic and lived body to the self and to society. As these knowledge bases encounter each other, new configurations of technology, capital, and the body are forged. I believe that the strength of new links and the persistence of old ones are related to religious heritage, cultural history, identity, and interpretations of liberal society, including concepts of rights and duties. Such social elements, along with the more technical aspects of tissue use, shape material practices in HBM technologies.

Because of the contingent and changing nature of such interactions, and because the various elements are not equivalent in terms of power or effect, practices are produced differently in different arenas. The chapters in this section show how elements such as religious ideas and heritage, political careers, economic interests, and historical changes in ideology or scientific knowledge can produce or change material practices around the body. These chapters ask, under what conditions can materials from the human body be used, and for which purposes?

Conceptions of the body have long been problematic. The relationship of identity to the physical body and of individual bodies to the social body are questions that have been resolved in various transient and often quixotic ways. Various cultural practices have been devised to distinguish persons from things, life from death, commodities from items that cannot be sold or exchanged. A number of new technologies bear witness to how these categories have been imploded: consider HBM as well as related technologies, including prosthetic devices, genetic engineering, and biohybrid human-synthetic devices.

But bodily boundaries have always been movable, and to move the boundary means to change ideas about bodily inviolability. The growing number of social scientists writing about the body in late twentieth-century capitalism tend to assume a generalized cultural resistance to the fragmentation of bodies, insisting that using bodily materials violates social norms. Such works rightly mark changes in the relation of the body to technology, but in doing so they make the mistake of presuming the existence of an original, natural, and authentic body. If they are correct to suggest that contemporary technologies violate a universal notion of bodily integrity, and that this violation is consistent across cultures, then there must be processes of cultural accommodation or resistance to deal with such sweeping transformations. Exactly how would these transformations occur while appearing not to violate cultural norms (or what we like to think are norms)? What about local conditions, cultures, and histories that affect not only responses to uses of the body but the forms of technologies and their related infrastructures?

Do cultural norms about the body exist unchanged? For centuries dead bodies have been dissected, dismembered, and distributed to multiple sites. All sorts of body parts have been displayed and traded as relics and teaching tools, collected as curios, used for research or healing preparations. While providing some historical background, chapters 2 and 3 consider the question, if bodily fragmentation has been going on for centuries, how has it been allowed to proceed, and what are the cultural byproducts?

Chapter 4 discusses legal constructions and definitions and shows how prevailing ideas and practices surrounding the treatment of body parts can be displaced or reinterpreted by competing claims and rights. Such claims may concern law enforcement, opportunities for scientific research, or the furthering of other social interests.[1]

Chapter 5 shows that there is, indeed, symbolic discontent over some uses of the body. But there need not be consensus on the nature or value of things, even things taken from the human body. In fact, public disputes become one way through which to deal with other social conflicts.

Repulsion and wonder as responses to various uses of the body coexist within countries, groups, and religious traditions. In none of the historical uses do I find evidence that there has ever been a unified reaction for or against a practice. Rather, esteem or disgust and the value assigned to body parts are viewed differently under different conditions, at different times, and among different groups. To suggest there is a homogenous medical community that stands apart from a homogenous society risks essentializing the identities of individuals and groups in societies in a way that anthropologists have long recognized will simply not hold.

Two

Animation and Regeneration

The Meaning of Death and the
Use of Body Materials in History

The body has long been a site for disputes about sacredness, scientific progress, and state sovereignty as they confront autonomy and personal control. Examining these disputes from a historical perspective, one sees that social and legal definitions of life and death change over time and that notions of what constitutes appropriate treatment of the body can be interpreted to suit specific purposes.

I find it curious, then, that many contemporary writings about the body refer to "traditional values" when discussing its appropriate handling. Social science and bioethics writings about organ transplantation in particular suggest that using body parts for any purpose is universally and uniformly taboo. Such notions derive in large part from religious (primarily western Christian) and legal imagery of the body as a temple, as a sacred vessel or locus of sanctity, or as an inalienable being—in other words, incapable of being considered an object.[1]

Other observers of economic and social conditions at the end of the millennium suggest that the body is becoming fragmented and commodified as never before and that this is a new phenomenon brought about solely by twentieth-century technological inventions and the postmodern condition. To state these ideas in an extreme form, flesh becomes commercial and the body dissolves as our identities are challenged by new technologies.

Upon examination, however, such abstract generalizations fall apart. The collection, use, and even sale of human remains are not new. In fact, for centuries the body—and, more specifically, substances removed from the dead body—has existed in various property-like states. So while some people are repulsed by the idea that human bodies are nothing more than organic objects, much less objects that can be mined as commercial resources, there are innumerable examples throughout history in which bodily materials have been used as exchangeable goods for healing, research, or profit. This is not to say that there was no resistance to such uses; rather, it shows that ideas and responses to various uses of human bodies are not so homogenous as sometimes presumed.[2]

At the heart of the dilemma is the question of whether removed parts of human bodies are things or if they retain some characteristic of personhood. This is important because access and rights to objects, as well as the ways in which we talk about and relate to them, operate under rules and practices distinct from those of inviolable persons (even dead ones), for whom societies have devised a variety of rituals, rules, and practices. What complicates the already prickly question of a body's status are uncertainties about the connection between animation and the body, particularly whether some form of life might remain in the organic body after death. If so, does it carry the identity of the person who has died? In Germany, as elsewhere, there is a long history of preoccupation with continued animation in the dead body. Such unresolved issues are being challenged by twentieth-century technologies that enable life to continue, but only in intimate connection with machines.

My point here is that the boundaries of human and nonhuman, living and dead, natural and technological are managed in order to rectify perceptions of bodily violation with certain desired outcomes. In this way new cultural mechanisms are devised that allow certain practices to proceed while appearing to sustain other cultural interests or virtues. Definitions of bodily inalienability and integrity can be modified in interaction with shifts in the values of scientific progress or altruism. For example, with the endorsement of legal, religious, and social institutions, doctors can enter bodies and treat tissues and organs like objects while maintaining fidelity to other interests, such as a patient's right to receive the best available medical care. Under certain conditions, then, the violation of a body's physical boundaries and sacrilege to sacred human remains can be reinterpreted as a sacrifice or gift that enables life to continue for someone else in need. I am less interested, therefore, in whether infractions of traditional beliefs are being committed or whether the body is more or less commodified than it was before than I am in the conditions under which definitions of bodily violation change.

The Body at Death

To learn how understandings of the body have changed over time and in different settings, one needs to look at burial practices and representations of death.[3] Since Arnold Van Gannep's (1909/1960) early work on rites of passage, anthropologists have been intrigued by mourning, body handling, and burial customs. In their studies of various cultures, Maurice Bloch and Jonathan Parry (1982), Robert Hertz (1907/1960), and Peter Metcalf and Richard Huntington (1979) have found patterns indicating that certain mortuary rituals deal with the liminality and uncertainty that arise when a member of society dies.

Hertz points out that the treatment of the corpse is not determined so much by the fate of the soul as by the nature of society itself and the way in which it manages social roles. Just as disposing of the body requires certain methods, the loss of a person from a group requires specific methods to reorder social relationships. After all, a societal member is "a social being grafted upon the physical being" (Hertz 1907/1960: 77). Certain rituals are thus devised to facilitate the disaggregation of social roles from this physical being, and other rituals create a new role for the dead person in a different sphere of existence. Disposal of the physical body can then be completed in a way consistent with society's beliefs about the body, the soul or identity, and regeneration or continuity. Because many societies consider the period immediately after death to be dangerous and uncertain, it is important to have rites that transfer the identity of the person peacefully but completely from one order into the next. Finally, to help survivors deal with the loss, societies have rites to reorder roles for those left behind.

It is important to note that similar customs may have different meanings and that mortuary practices are connected with beliefs about both material and immaterial parts of the person. For example, both Debbora Battaglia (1992, 1993) and Beth Conklin (1995) describe ritual cannibalism, in which the bodies of the dead are consumed as a way of simultaneously mourning and memorializing the dead. Battaglia (1993) suggests that, among the Sabarl Islanders of Melanesia, bodies are consumed as a collective project of forgetting. In contrast, the Wari' of Brazil also consume the dead but do so to affirm ideas of the regeneration of the natural human-animal order as expressed in Wari' myth and cosmology (Conklin 1995).

Setting aside the structuralist-functionalist nature of Hertz's argument and the fact that he studied small and what he assumed to be homogenous societies, I think that it is important to consider his points. Societies do order time and space in the death process through rituals and beliefs. While beliefs cannot be called "agreed upon and consistent," there are certain general trajectories that the dying are expected to follow. Disruption of these anticipated patterns calls for a response of some sort, either by resisting the disruption or accommodating oneself to it by modifying or reinterpreting the rituals.

In contemporary industrial societies, most people die in the hospital amid a variety of technologies that alter the dying process. New resuscitative techniques and official designation of new states (in particular, brain death) have changed the timing, recognition of cues, and procedures of the dying process. The body has been proclaimed dead, but it has not "died." Older rituals and staging of transformation to a different status have been modified as a result. In some societies, however, changes in the status of the dead, who is in charge of handling them, and how they are treated have caused considerable uproar.

I discuss changes in such routines in later chapters; but to understand differences in treatment of the dead body, one should examine the rituals that take place after the cadaver leaves the hospital. In contemporary Germany, 60 to 70 percent of bodies are cremated, so many that some people are concerned about the related air pollution (*Der Spiegel* 1995a). When a body is buried, the plot is not permanent; rather, it is leased for about twenty years. Coffins are made of simple wood, and bodies are not embalmed. They are allowed to disintegrate and disseminate into the earth naturally: dust to dust. Family members are often buried in the same plot, so the bones literally mingle with the bones of the ancestors. It is common to find bits of bone in the cemetery that have risen to the surface after years of digging up and reusing graves. One might argue, then, that Germans should have little objection to removing bits of tissue before the body is either burned or disintegrates.

Compare Germany with the United States, where bodies are preserved, beautified, sealed in steel and concrete, or placed in mausoleums. During the 1970s, 92 percent of American burials were earth burials, and 78 percent involved a full funeral and a viewing of the body (Pine 1975). Since then, the number of cremations has increased to 18 percent, although some regions in the south report only 3 percent. Of those bodies not cremated, more than 90 percent are embalmed (Iserson 1994: 224).

It is rare in Germany to view the body at memorial services. Respondents, however, told me that it is common to keep photographs of the dead together in the home and to make visits to the cemetery or otherwise memorialize a person's death at certain times. Graves are well kept, often decorated with hedges or flowers. The national holiday *Totensontag* is another way in which the dead are remembered; grave flowers are sold in the markets, special church services held, and people encouraged to visit the graves of friends and family. Thus, as the body slowly disappears, the person is commemorated and her presence kept alive through ritual acts that are separate from the body itself.

American customs of handling the dead suggest a desire to make the individual's corporeal existence permanent but in a way that seems less preoccupied with bodily integrity or fragmenting than with creating a solid form that endures. After all, embalming involves disembowelment, fills the body with toxic chemicals, and replaces or fills in features with cosmetic devices. Ritual disposal becomes a translation, much like the conversion of remains to relics in antiquity, with this difference: while the body is preserved as a permanent memorial in the ground, it is often not revered to the same extent or even usually remembered with visits or attention. There are few rituals of ongoing commemoration, except among certain religious and ethnic groups or within family traditions. Still, American customs reflect the belief that, even in death, property can be owned. Each individual has his own place for eternity; this is his memorial. In contrast to the Wari' and the Sabarl cultures, commemorations are made with mortar and stone. Headstones, statues, and gravesites are the depositories for memory that permit those left behind to forget.[4]

Philippe Ariès (1981) and Sabine Helmers (1989), among others, provide a number of examples of representations of sexuality and fertility in mortuary rituals and memorials. The implication is that many societies see death as a source of life. Aside from the literal interpretation of generation out of decay, there is a sense in which people deny the final nature of death by proclaiming it a new beginning. This is an important theme in the use of human materials for therapy, as later chapters will show.

Death as a Process: Animation and Material Continuity

In western societies, ideas about regeneration and the natural cycle of death into life are rooted in early Christian thinking, which had much to say about the locus of the soul or self in the physical body and what happens to the body after death. Central to the tenets of the Roman Catholic church, particularly through the first five centuries A.D., was the belief in the eventual resurrection of the intact, complete, and identical body after death.

The problem of how such bodily reassembly could occur was the subject of furious debate. What happens after death to body parts discarded during life, such as fingernails and foreskins? What happens to martyrs whose bodies have been torn apart by animals? What if they were eaten and digested? The apostle Paul, Justin Martyr, and other early Christian leaders were clear that bodies would rise with organs intact and flaws repaired (Bynum 1995a: 29). This undoubtedly helped early Christians deal with questions of how the pious who were tortured, burned, or mutilated could be resurrected with an uncorrupted body after death.[5]

Carolyn Walker Bynum, in her important work on the nature of human physical remains and the soul in early Christian beliefs (1990; 1995a, b), suggests that, while such ideas may seem bizarre to us, they must be taken seriously because they reflect the material ways in which people thought about the body and personhood. Today many people presume that the nature of the self in relation to the body was fundamental to the establishment of Christian doctrine. Bynum, however, argues that there was more concern about how parts of the body related to the whole being—that is, how they would be reintegrated after death. A great deal of anxiety focused on dismemberment and separation of parts from the whole body, but the real conceptual block was digestion: if bodies were digested, they would be absorbed into the eater's body, meaning that there might be too much for God to re-assemble. Even more troubling was the possibility that such absorption might represent a transmigration of souls (Bynum 1995a: 32).[6] The idea of a physical resurrection, then, answered concerns of the day: to rise with our bodies and its parts intact was a victory over digestion, dissemination, and assimilation into another form as much as a victory over death.

I suggest that early Christians may have been only partly concerned with transformation; the Bible promises something better: "So is the resurrec-tion of the dead. It is sown a perishable body, it is raised an imperishable body. . . . The trumpet will sound and the dead will be raised imperishable, and we shall be changed" (I Corinthians 15:42–52; all biblical quotations refer to the New American Standard Version unless otherwise noted). Rather, their fear may have related to an unanticipated event of dissemination that deviates from the promised or expected conversion.

By the twelfth and thirteenth centuries, new ideas about individual iden-tity and selfhood were percolating, including the belief that the material body was necessary to a notion of self. But it was not until the fourteenth cen-tury that Thomas Aquinas began to connect the notion of soul with identity and body in a way that could better satisfy questions of personal survival and the continuity of an individual's identity. His theory of hylomorphism maintained that only some bodily matter was soul-formed—that is, both physical and immaterial, imbued with and formed by the soul. Furthermore, the soul, which carried the specificity of each person, could activate matter to become that person's body at the time of resurrection. This certainly helped to resolve concerns about what happens at death to body bits that are removed from the body during life; most, he explained, are not soul-formed. This was a victory over dualism, which was later to be partly dis-mantled by Descartes's split of mind from body.

Another aspect of the relation of organic matter to the persistence of self after death was bodily experience during life. In particular, the act of incor-porating Christ's body through the Eucharist was based on the belief that the human body would be made whole and holy through Christ and would therefore be protected from decay. Christ himself appeared in bodily form after his death, even eating and drinking, proving both the bodily nature of

God and the physical nature of the body after death. Interestingly, in German the words of Jesus in the Eucharist are quite literal: "this is my body which is broken for you" (Luke 19:22). Although today the word *Leib* means "body," *Laib* was also used for "body" in early modern German; the words even sound the same. The literal meaning of *Laib* is "loaf," as in a loaf of bread. Thus, the body and the bread are both life-sustaining substances, the body both locus and instrument for redemption, a theme that recurs in organ transplantation. As I show later in this chapter and in chapters on procurement practice, the redemptive value of physical remains from the body can have much to do with the lived experience of the person who occupied and used it.

Exactly when does life—in whatever form—leave the cadaver? There are distinct differences in opinion among European regions and societies. According to Katherine Park (1995), southern European texts indicate a belief in an almost instantaneous change from the animated state of life to the inanimate state of death; the soul escapes the body and is no longer identified with the physical remains. Iconography in Italy depicts the dead as souls in purgatory separated from their bodies rather than bodies in a state of continued animation. Tomb sculptures in southern Europe carved during this time (approximately the thirteenth through the fifteenth centuries) show the intact body as it would have appeared in life—as though it were merely discarded rather than continuing to suffer (Park 1995: 125; see also Peters 1924, Schaefer 1920). This could help explain why dissection practices were accepted relatively easily in Italian centers of medicine compared to those in northern Europe.

According to Park, northern Europeans believed that the immaterial form of the self remained connected to the body for some period after death, slowly fading over time. In Germany, Britain, and France, people believed that death was a gradual process corresponding to the decay of the corpse, thought to be about one year (Park 1995: 114). Their preoccupation with the phases of decomposition was related to beliefs that a form of animated self remained in the body. Tomb sculptures found in Germanic territories show bodies with snakes and worms eating the entrails, but the body is usually standing or moving out of the grave. An etching from Berlin probably made between 1480 and 1490 shows a cadaver in this condition, emphasizing the process of decay (see figure 2.1).

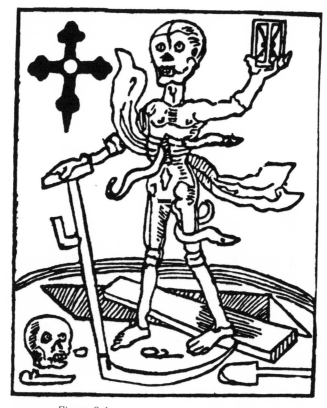

_____ *Figure 2.1* _____

Leichengift

Source: Peters (1924), 135.

Note the prominent poison mark in the left corner of figure 2.1. In German mythology, the existence of *Leichengift,* or poison from cadavers, referred to the toxic byproducts of putrefaction. It was an element of danger or taboo (Helmers 1989). The corpse, then, was both animated and contaminating. This dual nature of vitality, with its potential to give life or to endanger it, continues to be a theme in the use of tissues from the dead. Cadaver tissues and organs can substitute for malfunctioning parts in the new host and thus be life-saving. At the same time, they can carry infectious agents and molecules that cause damaging tissue reactions. In fact, the greatest clinical problem with transplanted organs and tissues is blocking the infective and antigenic agency of grafted tissue.

People believed that cadavers could be quite active: they could perspire, bite, turn over, gnaw their limbs or shrouds, continue to grow hair and nails, and perform other bodily functions. This notion was codified in Germanic law until late in the seventeenth century. For example, the principle of *Bier-recht* or *Bahrrecht* held that the body of a murder victim bled in the presence of the murderer. This sign could be used as legal evidence to identify and convict the perpetrator (Ariès 1981, Linke 1986, Schaefer 1920). Thus, the dead body retained certain powers and capabilities that not only implied a transitional state of animation but lent the cadaver a type of agency in human affairs.

In sum, death was not believed to be complete until the body was fully decomposed. This state of continued animation caused a great deal of anxiety in terms of knowing when a person was actually dead. A preoccupation with *Scheintod* (apparent death; the idea that persons who appeared dead were in fact alive) existed in Germany from the fourteenth until the mid-nineteenth century, reaching a peak in the seventeenth and again in the late eighteenth century.

While apparent-death stories circulated throughout northern Europe, in Germany they reached near-panic proportions. It is not surprising, then, that the first funeral homes were probably developed in Germany. These *vitae dubiae azilia* (shelters for doubtful life) appeared in Munich, Weimar, Berlin, and Mainz between 1791 and 1818. They were used as a place where bodies could be stored and observed for several days to ensure that they were, indeed, dead. A new profession was born as specialists were called upon to determine death and watch over the dead bodies.

Burials during panics about Scheintod created innovations in practices, material culture, and markets. Special coffins were devised with signal mechanisms in case the person awoke, and various devices were sold to detect life at the gravesite. The manner of wrapping and preparing bodies changed. The time between death and burial increased because more individuals instructed survivors to leave their bodies untouched (unembalmed and undissected) lest they were still alive (Ariès 1981). Culture making was linked with profit making as public concerns influenced material social practices.

Martin Pernick (1988) argues that scientific discoveries in experimental physiology and resuscitation techniques had much to do with the concern over apparent death. He points out that controversy peaked between the mid-eighteenth and the mid-nineteenth centuries, correlating with key discoveries in experimental physiology. For example, in 1774, electricity was first used to resuscitate a human, transforming scientific ideas about the body's ability to reanimate. The experiment suggested that a vital force might exist that could simply be restarted. Instruments were designed to check for signs of life, and elaborate tests were created to measure activity in dead bodies. For the first time, technological innovations enabled the detection of muscular contractions and a heartbeat that persisted some time after death. Such innovations provided explanations (or at least better observations) for phenomena, but ultimately they created even greater ambiguity about when death actually occurs.

As Pernick rightly points out, uncertainties about the body at death have much to do with public perceptions of science and medical expertise. There was a growing faith in not only the ability of science but also its role in answering important questions of the day. Otherwise, there would have been little support for such inquiry, and discoveries would not have had the sort of effect Pernick and others have described.

Clearly, mortuary ritual, including the physical handling of the body, mourning customs, legal conventions, and economic innovations, changes as it interacts with prevailing cultural and scientific beliefs. Yet it is important to remember that there were class differences in the ways in which human remains were handled and technological innovations were applied. Special coffins, devices, and handling were made only for the rising bourgeoisie and the wealthy. Paupers were thrown into shallow mass graves, often with no formal funeral ceremony (Laqueur 1983). Few poor people were attended at death; rarely did anyone detect life signs or attempt resuscitation.

Sacred Commodities: Trade in Bodily Materials

All this attention paid to the body, including changes in ritual disposal designed to deal with its indeterminate status, made it a cultural object open to a variety of transactions. Cadavers and body parts were used as symbolic elements (relics), knowledge-producing objects (anatomical specimens), and objects of commerce and other forms of exchange. Thus, body parts from the dead existed simultaneously as sacred remains and vehicles for income. For example, among the German aristocracy from the twelfth through the sixteenth centuries, it was desirable to have one's body parts buried in different territories. This was particularly important during the Crusades, when many soldiers died on pagan soil and wanted their bodies to be moved to their Christian homelands. It became common practice to have bodies divided—that is, dismembered so that various parts could be buried in different places. The practice was known as *mos teutonicus,* or "the German custom" (Binski 1996). It necessitated boiling the cadavers or separating flesh from bones since Germans did not traditionally embalm, although Italians and others did. Outside of Germany, the practice was considered barbaric; indeed, Pope Boniface VIII officially condemned the practice in 1299. Nevertheless, since family members and individuals were expected to pray at the burial sites of higher-ranking individuals under whose protection they existed, the German elite soon realized that dividing the remains allowed the deceased to profit from prayers at several shrines, assuring his position in eternity. Thus, the pope's official interdiction had the inverse effect of making the practice even more desirable because only the highest-ranking members of society could get an exception to the rule after 1300 (Brown 1981). At the same time, the practice enabled communities to draw visitors and trade by claiming a piece of an illustrious individual. In these ways, dead bodies continued to serve the souls of the deceased as well as the interests of communities.

Even greater value could be generated in body parts by producing relics made from practically any remains of a saint or martyr. Relics had no value as body parts per se; but if people believed that a certain person had a special status during life or even after death, then special treatment was called for. In his enlightening study of the culture and politics of relics, Patrick Geary notes that their value could only be created through their transition from ordinary body remains to venerated object via public rituals (1986: 178). These body bits were seen as security deposits left by saints as guarantees of their continued interest in earthly affairs after their death. Communities benefited from protection by virtue of the relics' presence. More directly, they profited from pilgrimages that drew trade and commerce to relic sites (Geary 1986: 180; Park 1995: 112). Cult centers, competing for the devotion of the faithful, depended on rare and important relics to draw pilgrims. A thriving relic trade and methods to authenticate the source and efficacy of relics were two cultural innovations that emerged from the way in which these particular body parts were valued (Geary 1978).

The value of relics fluctuated over time and according to various social and political conditions. During periods of weak central power, relics were a crucial substitute for public authority and a source of protection. The church or royal authorities also centralized control over sacred elements as a means of regulating access to certain sites for political purposes.

When bodies—especially dead ones—develop property or commodity-like characteristics, who or what has jurisdiction over them? Laws specifying rights and protection of the dead have existed for several centuries in Germany. Legal concepts of *Störung der Totenruhe* (disturbing the dead) were significant in early legal codes and figure prominently in German folklore as well. The related concept of *Totensorgerecht* deals with rights to and control over the dead body itself. My field notes are peppered with this term. Study participants called it a centuries-old concept, although I was unable to find its roots in legal documents. Nevertheless, almost everyone knew the term, explaining it as both a duty and a right to have the body and care for it according to traditional funerary practice or the wishes of the deceased.

Interestingly, several respondents who opposed having a law allowing bodies to be used for research and therapy without family permission cited Sophocles' play *Antigone*. In the play, the king, Creon, declares that the body of Antigone's brother should remain unburied since he was considered an enemy of the state. Antigone fights for her right to bury her brother according to custom. The respondents linked Antigone's impulse toward duty and care of the body to the German tradition of Totensorgerecht. As far as they were concerned, the conflict between private duty and the state's claim to authority over its subjects' bodies was being played out on the stage of late twentieth-century politics.

Bodies of Knowledge: Dissections and Collections

The conflict between private and public responsibility extends to the history of anatomical dissection. While dissection appeared to violate taboos against opening dead bodies, social relations among healers, the church, and sovereign authorities were creating an environment in which it could occur. As dissection became routine, further changes in legal conventions and bodily practices were introduced.

The use of bodies for dissection and anatomical displays in Europe is well documented.[7] Anxiety created by the uncertainty of death, dying, and disease in increasingly secularized societies created a need to seek alternative accounts for phenomena. The growing practice of opening bodies under the direction of medical practitioners demystified the body and provided new explanations. Thus, physicians became an alternative to clergy for distinguishing natural from mystical phenomena.[8]

Contradicting historians who argue that there were strong social and church taboos against opening dead bodies, Park (1994), among others, points out that dissections were also conducted for private clients and often requested by dying patients or their families if the cause of illness was uncertain. Throughout the Middle Ages, Christians believed in physical markings of spirituality, and this belief allowed the opening and dismembering of bodies. For instance, hearts of saints were opened to discover the name of Jesus written upon them or a cross emblazoned upon the flesh.

By the sixteenth century, however, dissection was also used as an extreme form of punishment, inflicted after death as a final insult to and total destruction of a body that had offended the sovereignty and sovereign laws (Foucault 1979). Bodies of executed criminals were handed over to anatomists or barber-surgeons, who performed dissections in public. "A punishment worse than death" was linked with the increasing demand for dissection material for medical purposes, forming a tie between the medical profession and the judiciary. The misfits and less valued individuals in society could thus not only be punished and eliminated but be put to good use by medical professionals who benefited from their increased knowledge of human anatomy. This theme recurred under Nazism, as I discuss in chapter 3, but arguments from this utilitarian perspective continue today—for example, in the outrage over executing criminals in China expressly for organ donation.

Dissection was defended in terms of the medical benefits: the ends justify the means. Knowledge, techniques, and procedures of dissection led to an established field of inquiry through which physical structures could be viewed and disease processes seen in relation to these structures rather than understood as external or metaphysical events. Stanley Tambiah (1990) asserts that this area of inquiry received political sanction, although corresponding scientific investigations of the human mind and behavior did not, remaining matters of the soul and therefore of the church. The power of dissection as a punishment, which was built upon the idea of the final destruction of identity, bodily integrity, and the soul, had thus generated a new set of debates and social arrangements among the church, the state, and the growing field of medicine.

The growing demand for cadavers could not be sated by the supply of criminal bodies alone. At the same time public protests against "mutilation of the dead" were increasing, sometimes preventing collection of the corpse (Richardson 1989, Rupp 1992). As anatomists began to establish schools, competition for bodies became more heated; and scarcity of supply meant that corpses acquired money value. By the late seventeenth century, agents of physicians began approaching prisoners to barter their own corpses for money to pay their prison expenses. Additionally, fees were paid to individuals who robbed graves, stole bodies from poorhouses, or killed marginal members of society. The fresher the corpse, the more valuable it was; and rare or exotic bodies, such as the congenitally malformed or giants, fetched large sums of money for private collections.[9]

With a growing and lucrative market, grave robbing and cadaver supply evolved into a trade. Areas with a nearby anatomy school or university were particularly subject to extensive grave robbing. Paupers' graves were vulnerable because they were shallow and often left open until they were full of bodies (Laqueur 1983). Legally, corpses were not considered to be property; therefore, removal from graves was not considered to be theft. While police did pursue resurrectionists, they were often instructed not to be overzealous and to turn a blind eye to robbing from burial grounds of the poor.

Most people were well aware of these activities and were concerned about the fate of their own and their loved ones' bodies. Called villains and thieves, resurrectionists were dragged through the streets and beaten in protest. Public demonstrations peaked by the late 1700s and early 1800s.[10] They took place throughout northern Europe, although Britain was the first country to pass a comprehensive anatomy law in 1832. This was also the high point of the Scheintod panics in Germany, indicating not only fear of being buried alive but also worry about the body's fate after death. The effect of dissection on physical resurrection was a central concern.

Questions about anatomists' disrespectful treatment of bodies were also raised. People suspected that women's bodies were subjected to voyeurism and necrophilia and that leftover body parts were fed to animals. An investigation of one body-snatching incident in England reported that candles and soap were made from the remains (Richardson 1989: 97).

Resistance to and protest against dissection, grave robbing, and other practices involving the invasion of dead bodies was not necessarily based on moral grounds alone (Ariès 1981, Park 1995, Richardson 1989, Schaefer 1920). Nor could it have been entirely based on particular religious beliefs, especially after the late sixteenth century, when religious sects proliferated and dogmas split into many versions.[11] Rather, the practices spoke to the lack of control over the body and the power of the state—or other authorities, such as scientific experts—to make decisions about what were commonly held to be private matters. It was the manner and source of procurement as much as the fact of their use that created problems around the use of dead bodies.

The Healing and Regenerative Power of Human Material

Once collected, cadavers yielded scientific knowledge and products that could be collected, preserved, examined, and exchanged for a variety of research and teaching purposes in the growing field of medicine. But cadaver parts were also used more directly for medicinal purposes. References in legal and medical documents indicate that cadaver parts were widely believed in Germany to have healing and regenerative powers. Cadavers were included in the healing pharmacopoeia in many parts of northern Europe during the sixteenth and seventeenth centuries. For example, perspiration from newly dead persons was said to heal tumors, and the hand of a corpse, especially if still warm, cured epilepsy. Drugs were also made from the fat or flesh of cadavers.

Certain types of cadavers were considered to be particularly valuable sources of therapeutic treatments. For example, the use of blood as a healing agent was common in folklore, but emphasis was on the rejuvenating power of pure sources, such as blood from virgins or children. On the other hand, Paracelsus, the German mystic physician, used mummia (an extract from cadavers) for healing but insisted that it was only effective when derived from the bodies of those who had died unnatural or traumatic deaths. The touch of a recently hanged person was said to cure skin ailments, goiter, ulcers, and cancers (Richardson 1989: 53). A German Lutheran doctor in the late seventeenth century had a recipe for regenerative divine water that required cutting the body of someone who had died a violent death (but was in good health) into small pieces and reducing it to a liquid (Ariès 1981: 358).[12]

Some of the oldest monastic healing texts describe blood remedies for certain illnesses. Blood from corpses, especially from those who died a violent death, was said to alleviate pain and cure chronic illnesses (Ankert 1918, Dölger 1926). Executioners were allowed to sell the blood of criminals upon execution as late as the nineteenth century. Ulrike Linke (1986: 230) reports regular requests for blood as an ingredient in medical remedies: "High and mighty noble, especially honorable judge! Having learned that the execution shall proceed at this time, I hereby request permission to catch the blood of the delinquent, since I need the same for very useful medicines in our pharmacy (J. Leitmeritz, July 21, 1729)."

Here is another example of the public demand for human blood:

I attended the public execution of a female prisoner at Göttingen. It was done with a sword. When the head was severed from the body, and the fountain of blood sprang up, the populace broke through the square formed by the Hannover Schützen, rushed upon the scaffold and possessed itself of the blood of the dead woman, collecting it and dipping white cloths in it. . . . To my horrified question I got the answer that the blood was applied for the cure of epilepsy." (communication of Attorney-General Woyotasch of Marienwerder, August 1892, quoted in Linke [1986: 235])

The source of the cadaver and the manner of death are of considerable interest. Violent or sudden death might rule out the possibility of infectious or chronic illnesses that could be passed on or otherwise contaminate the person receiving cadaver materials. Similarly, a young person or virgin is arguably less likely to have degenerative diseases or to have been exposed to certain undesirable illnesses. Documents from Berlin and Jena indicate that higher prices were paid for blood from virgins and children and that blood from Jews fetched a far lower price (Jaeckel 1986, Strack 1909). Sudden death, however, often meant execution of a criminal or social outcast, a person one would normally not want near—much less on or in—one's body. In addition, we do not know if higher prices for young sources represented rarity or belief in effectiveness. There is some contradiction, then, between the qualities of the person-as-source and the quality and effectiveness of parts of her body as healing agents.

The choice of human rather than animal or plant sources otherwise available in the pharmacopeia indicates a nexus of material and symbolic concerns. Animal and plant sources were used for the majority of ailments because they were readily available and there were few moral injunctions against their use. Such sources, however, were even more prized for food and work. In contrast, the bodies of criminals were certainly available, particularly after public executions, as the example I have quoted illustrates. The state soon stepped in to control the supply of these valued sources, allowing only certain medical practitioners and apothecaries access to the remains.

It is not clear if human and nonhuman sources were considered to be equivalent or interchangeable, so we are left asking, For which conditions were human sources in particular seen to be effective healing tools? What was it about human materials that was believed to be effective? I suggest that the unresolved questions of animation in the body allows for the possibility that a lingering vitality, when transferred to the user, had regenerative capability. Thus, while blood or other material from a pure source was thought to be cleansing and healing, the image of innocence and purity may not have been as important as the transformative power of the material itself. That is, the value of the material as a curative agent may have depended more on the belief that organic human matter was still animate than on specific biological or medicinal properties of the tissue. In the process, the transfer of a human vital force could be seen as a parallel process to resurrection—the "gift of life," as we say today.

Popular beliefs that cadavers could continue to perform normal bodily functions reinforced the idea that corpses maintain a type of vitality. While this had significance in terms of regenerative capabilities, the idea of using materials or parts from dead bodies made it important to determine whether or not a cadaver still had sensibility—that is, whether or not the body part maintained a connection to its previous owner. Dresden physician Christian Friedrich Garmann insisted that some force exists that connects body parts, wherever they are. He reported the case of a German who had a nose removed from a living person and grafted on to replace his own, lost in battle.

The nose is said to have stayed in place until it quite suddenly rotted. It was later discovered that the nose "died" and decomposed at the same time that its original donor died, convincing Garmann that corpses do indeed have sensibility.

Such ideas about continued animation and sensibility may seem quaint to us today, but similar ideas and concerns appear in contemporary narratives from and about recipients of transplanted organs. While I was doing research in the United States, I often heard reports of organ recipients who had developed strange tastes in food or habits or had gained certain insights or knowledge about the donor that they attributed to characteristics implanted with the organ (see also Sharp 1995). Lesley Sharp (1995) recounts fascinating stories from recipients who reported changes in their own sense of personhood after receiving someone else's organ. This becomes a conundrum of continued animation: the perceived vitality of the tissue plays a role in its usefulness and thus its value; but if another persona seems to be implanted along with the tissue, even more complex issues arise.

Many Germans with whom I spoke were quite clear that personhood existed down to the cellular level. For some, this was the primary reason why they opposed moving any tissue from one person to another. As one respondent put it, "every cell in our bodies is *us*—every cell is part of our identity, which does not belong in someone else's body" (f.n., January 1994). Another person believed that body parts were central to each individual's identity: "organs belong to the human creature as an integral component of his individuality and personhood" (f.n., May 1994).

Postmortem: Use Value, Exchange, and Control of Bodily Materials

As I have shown, there are material consequences to prevailing beliefs: political, economic, technological, and other interests can affect and be affected by theories about the body and personhood. In addition, the production of cultural products from the body, including medicinal therapies, relics, anatomical specimens, and work models for medical students, involve several forms of transmutation. Organic decaying tissue can be preserved or processed to become a healing tool or a sacred political and social symbol. The dead human body can become a means for producing or disseminating scientific knowledge and an object with exchange value. But for such uses to proceed, biological remains must come to be seen as commodities. Human bodies must be culturally reclassified as something other than precious human remains, or they must be transformed into something that can exist in another category. This requires a cultural mechanism that makes certain uses appear to be consistent with other cultural values, such as the pursuit of knowledge, or the addition of symbolic or other capital for the good of society as a whole.

Practices and discourses that surround the materials reveal ways in which the relation of identity to biology varies according to use and desired effect. For example, a skull used for teaching should be anonymous, divorced from its former identity. The source for that object—a criminal, a pauper, a nameless volunteer—is construed to have contributed something of value through her death. On the other hand, the skull of a saint needs to have its identity authenticated for the relic to have value as an exchange object or for its magical effect.

The value of things is related not only to their usability and exchangeability but also to their accessibility. Certain kinds of bodies were easier to use for both practical and cultural reasons, so they become candidates for use. The poor, people who had no family to carry out traditional funerary rituals or to protect the dead, and criminals were made available by the state with the sanction of the church and the additional incentive of economic gain under certain circumstances. In these cases, additional value was actually created through the act of bodily destruction after death.

Other forms of fragmenting and commodification of bodies, such as the mos teutonicus or the invention of relics, were treatments that operated on the bodies of privileged or distinct individuals. Division and relic preservation were fashionable customs through which privileged classes either circumvented the law for their own bodies or created new religious edicts that ultimately benefited merchant and wealthy classes.

In the process of being reclassified, taking on more or less value, the sources themselves can become transformed. Thus, diseased and dying bodies are regenerated at the same time that degenerate sources can themselves be redeemed. As Barleus said in 1632, "the criminal who had done so much harm to society, can now, after his death, be of great use to society" (Rupp 1992: 50). The ability and opportunity to turn social waste—useless human lives as well as human body byproducts—into something useful is a powerful transformation. Elsewhere, I have described the contemporary symbolic importance of using "good" sources as compared to "making something worthwhile out of worthless lives" (Hogle 1992, 1995b). What I observed about organ procurement in the United States was that donors who were prototypically "good" sources for tissue—people with safe lifestyles who were unlikely to be involved in crime or drugs, for example—were not necessarily best in terms of the overall procurement process. "Bad" persons—criminals, troubled youth, and other less desirable members of society—quite often became the actual donors out of the pool of potential ones. In other words, a "good" donor was not the same as a "good" donation. To illustrate, in one case a procurement coordinator discussed a donor who was labeled a juvenile delinquent:

> We see all the really bad cases—the dregs of humanity. It gets so depressing. I see donor work as more hopeful. Take that kid. Now his life was really worthless. . . . he just wasted his life. So he got himself shot up. Now his mother can say he donated his organs for other people. That's something she can say for the next thirty years—not "oh, he got shot up." (Hogle 1995b: 493)

Thus, one product of organ transplantation as a beneficial use of human bodies is a type of social redemption. Organ transplantation in the United States has also become a public symbol denoting that we are an altruistic society. For many, organ donation has become an act of commemoration as well as an attempt to assure some sort of material continuity.

There are other changes in material practices that contribute to cultural changes. Perceiving and using human bodies in a different way requires drawing upon an existing store of cultural knowledge and modifying it to produce new knowledge. New markets are created for otherwise unusable or unused goods. Entire industries spin off from the ability to find and use human material. New ways of thinking about the body and commerce have emerged. The creation and circulation of material value thus proceeds in connection with cultural profit in the sense of innovation and change (Gudeman 1992).

In sum, the use of bodies and their parts for healing, study, and exchange is not a new phenomenon in Germany or elsewhere. Nor are the various interpretations and reactions to these practices new, although they are historically distinct in Germany. Differing treatments of the body and its parts appear relatively acceptable and natural, macabre, or senseless based on various contexts and perspectives and, of course, on the manner in which the human sources were acquired. To some of us today, the thought of chopping up bodies for distribution throughout the country or preserving scabs from revered individuals in elegant reliquaries seems bizarre and perhaps perverse. To others, the suggestion that some people today refuse to donate their organs or accept organs from others because of vestigial Judeo-Christian beliefs promulgated as a response to first-century persecutions— an idea suggested by contemporary writers who assume universal and fundamental "cultural insistence on body inviolability"—seems equally naïve.

Still, contemporary views of bodily integrity, particularly at death, exhibit concerns similar to those existing in centuries past. The way in which boundaries of life and death are established; a certain repulsion at the opening and handling of the dead; fears about death and decay; and changing notions of identity, continuity, or transformation of self in the material body are all perplexities that affect conceptions of dead bodies and the proper way of handling them. But as chapter 3 will show, laws, customs, and even religious guidelines can be changed in unexpected ways to accommodate competing values and interests.

Three

Embodying National Identity

National Socialism and the Body

Just as cultural meanings surrounding the body change with historical, political, economic, and technological conditions, meanings are mutually constituted along with the creation of categories such as sacred remains, useful resources, waste, human person, or organic thing. As chapter 2 demonstrated, the ways in which such meanings and practices shift provide parameters for what is possible and allowable to do with human bodies and their parts.

I turn now to the most powerful example in German experience: the selected use and ultimate destruction of some bodies for the benefit of others under National Socialism. The joining of medical science, modernist technology, and antimodern ideology during the Fascist regime had devastating consequences when applied to the large-scale social projects of racial hygiene and euthanasia. National Socialist politics instituted a differential valuing of various types of humans so that certain humans could be considered experimental objects—too worthless to participate in a superior German society, yet quite valuable in the economics of science in service to the state. The history of medicine under National Socialism has had a far-reaching influence on medical practices today, initiating changes in legal codes and serving as a warning against abuses in medicine and scientific practice both in Germany and around the world.

The story is one in which national identity became quite literally

embodied, inscribed upon members who belonged and branded on the fore-
arms of those who did not. Three points are crucial to understanding the
impact of National Socialism on medical practice in Germany today: the myth
of a superior national biological and social body, the redefining as refuse of
those who did not belong, and the social and technical means to convert
refuse into a valuable resource for the good of the social body.

Under National Socialism, the word was made flesh as national identity
was tied to the physicality of society's members. Social problems were related to human vitality; the fitness of the nation was related to the fitness of
the individuals who constituted it. The German social body as a central image became the vehicle through which the modernist science of eugenics
was wedded to revitalized romantic notions of authentic German culture.[1]
The search to find scientific ways to identify, protect, and maintain
Germanness became a powerful political tool. Theories of racial hierarchies
were the foundation upon which science and the state together could
reconceptualize the value of human lives. The state thus became the arbi-
ter of the social good, creating racial hygiene programs not only to improve
the Aryan race but to destroy *lebensunwertes Lebens* (lives unworthy of living).

In this way, the health of the social body was assured by acting on the
bodies of individuals. The use or disposal of some bodies for the benefit of
others, however, required an institutionalized shift in the way in which certain bodies were viewed. The concept of inviolability of the body had to
change, and who had the right to use which bodies and for what purposes
had to be clarified. Unworthy lives were reconceptualized as waste, not even
human. But it was only by applying scientific knowledge, technologies, and
new techniques that such waste could be further converted into a valuable
resource. The development of the notion of a German social body is key to
understanding why contemporary uses of individual human bodies and the
employment of rational technoscientific approaches to improve the health
of the greater good—the societal body—are more problematic in Germany
than elsewhere.

The Social Body: Physical and Symbolic Codes
of Membership

In the first decades of the twentieth century, Germany was suffering from a dramatic increase in urban crowding, poverty, disease, alcohol-

ism, and other social changes caused by urbanization and industrialization as well as the tremendous loss of healthy young men during World War I. According to some scientists and social thinkers of the day, all that was left were people unfit to be German citizens. By this time, scientists were exploring the possibility of selecting desirable genetic traits. Applying scientific laws of biology and hygiene became the solution to preventing further degeneration of the German people and restoring the nation's hereditary fitness (Weindling 1989: 320). Biological approaches in policy initially aimed at reducing the number of alcoholics, derelicts, and mental incompetents through a combination of genetic selection and social mechanisms such as controlling individuals' lifestyles to prevent the reproduction of undesirable traits. The policies were known as *Rassenhygiene, Sozialhygiene,* and *Volkshygiene* (racial, social, and peoples' or population hygiene).

As Paul Weindling (1989) shows in his exhaustive study of scientific disciplines in early twentieth-century Germany, the concept of racial hygiene was rapidly popularized because it attracted the support of a wide variety of professional groups. For example, applying "scientific" methods to identifying degenerate and superior groups increased the professional stature of groups such as anthropologists, which had long been interested in classifying races by morphology and biology.[2] Likewise, physicians could expand the medical domain into social and economic areas by applying medical solutions to social problems. Between them, anthropological and medical approaches to racial hygiene formed a productive synthesis (Lifton 1986, Proctor 1988, Weindling 1989).

By the end of World War I, biological approaches were increasingly applied to groups rather than individuals through population and reproductive control and public surveillance using epidemiological techniques. Societies began to be defined in organicist terms—that is, understood as organisms subject to natural cycles of birth, maturity, and decay. Increasingly, biological terms and metaphors were applied to social and political concerns, culminating in the unique concept of the *Volkskörper* (literally, the body of the people, or society as a body). The nation was idealized as a highly integrated community, or *Volksgemeinschaft,* and represented the moral regeneration of family and *Volk*. Families were seen as elemental cells of the state organism, and the alarming decrease in family size (of the more desirable German citizens) was described as cellular degeneration (Weindling 1989: 291).

The individual body became an icon of national unity and productivity while contributing to the health and fitness of the German social body. Therefore, individual bodies had to stay healthy to keep the overall system going. Personal hygiene, fresh air, diet, sports, and behavioral control were seen as ways to build up the organic whole. Intimately related to this physical well-being was a renewal of spiritual vitality. *Völkisch* thinking was based on a romantic notion of spirituality connected to a cosmic vitality believed to be particular to Germans and containing mystical and occult elements from the "original" Germanic people. According to George Mosse (1964/1981), even Christianity had to be Germanized to allow *das Volk* to exercise a uniquely German set of ethical principles. Purity of spirit and body was paramount for descendants with the bloodlines of authentic Germans.[3]

It was equally important that German citizens be protected from invasions of infectious, unauthentic, or otherwise damaging agents. Protection from outside penetration became critical to the ongoing survival of the social body. This included protection from Jews, Communists, Gypsies, homosexuals, and others, who were often depicted in narratives and popular art as insects, rodents, or disease carriers infesting German society.[4] Thus, while earlier racial hygiene programs sought to eliminate impurities, the selection, separation, and ultimate mass murder of these groups sought to create a nonpermeable boundary that would prevent contamination.

Blood was a key symbol: "To us [the National Socialists] blood not only means something corporeal, but it is in a sense the soul, which has as its external field of expression the body" (Clauss 1936: 147). One racial hygiene society likened the losses of World War I to a body bleeding to death. Symbolically and literally, the purity of blood became central to establishing who belonged in the German body.

The popular nationalist slogan *Blut und Boden* (blood and soil) strengthened the connection between German heredity and homeland-as-body. Biological metaphors were linked with notions of belonging and rootedness to German lands. In this way, racial hygiene became a material way of forging a national identity. *Germanness* was defined with medical criteria that excluded outsiders and "primordialized" insiders.

To purify and protect the blood from outsiders, laws were established in the 1930s that forbade marriages between Aryans and non-Aryans, and pronatal policies were established to breed more desirable Germans. At the same time, sterilization of undesirable members of society prevented them from procreating. Selective euthanasia was another social-medical program instituted to improve the health of the social body. In addition to the "inferior" races, the mentally ill and congenitally deformed were systematically exterminated.

Eventually, epileptics, individuals with chronic inheritable diseases, and homosexuals were included in the list of unnecessary and burdensome people who cost society more than they were worth. The biological metaphor was extended to reconceptualize these humans as social waste. The Reich Health Council Circular of 1931 defines societal waste clearly:

> Thus in the name of the National Socialist "Third Reich" a medical doctor would have the following mission, in order to create a "new noble humanity": only those who can recover would be healed. The sick who cannot recover, however, are dead weight existences, human refuse, unworthy of living and unproductive. They must be destroyed and eliminated. (Dr. H. Moses, cited in Pross and Aly 1989: 92)

Euthanasia and large-scale extermination programs became the methods of excretion.

Waste into Useful Resource: Human Experimentation

While many humans were seen as social waste, they had considerable value as organic bodies. Government euthanasia, internment, and extermination programs allowed clinical and research physicians to use victims—and materials from their bodies—as resources for experimentation. The internment of thousands of humans created a controllable environment and easy access to research materials. As the authorities reasoned, these prisoners would die or be killed in any case; they had no power to object or interfere.

Researchers could use living prisoners to determine the metabolic and physiological effects of certain treatments. They could test solutions to immediate problems in military medicine or use organs and tissue from dead prisoners to demonstrate anatomical differences. Physicians were able to carry out elaborate experiments not otherwise possible, especially on such a large scale. Young physicians were encouraged to build their reputations by carrying out experiments on prisoners in the camps. They could thus simultaneously serve the cause and have a ready source of the raw materials required for finishing their medical study.[5] Josef Mengele, for example, collected and preserved organs for Otmar Verschuer of the Kaiser Wilhelm Institute für Anthropologie (KWI) as part of his *Habilitation,* or postdoctoral research (Kater 1987: 126). He went on to conduct the most extreme and inhumane of the medical experiments.

The ideal site for experiments, Auschwitz had been designed with a large clinic right next to a building where victims could be gassed after experimentation. Physicians and anthropologists selected research subjects when new interns arrived at the camp, sending those deemed suitable or medically or genetically interesting to the infamous Block 10, which housed the subjects of experiments. Twins were particularly interesting since they had similar tissue and blood types: physicians could study reactions to various bodily insults on one twin while using the other as a built-in control.

Many experiments tested human survivability under extreme physiological stress and were originally designed to benefit German soldiers during the war.[6] Nevertheless, investigations of organ function and disease processes had broader implications, influencing the development of fields such as immunology and surgery long after the war.

Of interest to the later development of tissue transplantation were tissue regeneration and grafting experiments. Researchers hoped that studies of the regeneration of bone, muscle, and nerve tissue would not only be helpful in treating soldiers' wounds but might reveal ways to grow or replace diseased tissue in civilian patients (Lifton 1986). While many of these trials seem bizarre or at least not well grounded in scientific theory, findings from some studies yielded data that have been used in tissue typing and wound healing research. At the time researchers had little understanding of immunology, so tissue grafting trials—particularly those performed on twins—provided entirely new data that would not have been obtainable otherwise.

There was a large program of bone grafting experiments carried on in the Ravensbrück camp for women. Bones of both lower legs were broken into several pieces with a hammer and repaired with bone chips from another subject. In other experiments, entire fibulae were excised and implanted into either another camp research subject or a soldier wounded in action. Some bone and tissue from prisoners were sent to Dr. Karl Gebhardt, professor of orthopedic surgery at the University of Berlin, where they were transplanted into patients at his clinic in Hohenlychen (Mitscherlich 1949).

The camps provided opportunities for German pharmaceutical companies to test experimental preparations, such as the new sulfa drugs. Numerous infections occurred as a result of tissue or bone removal, and infections were also induced to test medicines.

The Collectible Body: The Use of Body Materials for Display and Research

In additional to using living human bodies to conduct appalling experiments, researchers viewed these bodies as an inexpensive and readily available source of materials. Human tissue was removed for dissection and further experimentation and collected for demonstration and teaching purposes. Researchers turned to human sources to make tissue culture medium because, during wartime, it was easier to obtain and far more expendable than valuable animal meat. The *Schutztaffel*, or SS, a special military defense squadron, was responsible for acquiring materials for experiments, including the animal meat normally used to produce culture media. The chief SS physician at the Berlin Hygiene Institute found it very simple to replace that meat with human flesh. One witness described seeing four women's bodies removed. Then, a half-hour later, "the bodies came back to their place, but they were mutilated and had cut out of them large areas deep into the flesh" (Lifton 1986: 289). Inmates working in a lab had already suspected the change after noticing "in the culture media pieces of meat with hairless skin" (Langbein 1972: 398).

Physicians were fascinated by the possibility of collecting brains and skeletons representing different populations or various conditions. Samples could be prepared in clinics where people were being euthanized and either used within the clinic or sent to other central research institutes, such as the KWI in Berlin. Professor Hallervorden, of the institute's center for brain research, was delighted at the prospect of acquiring a large number of specimens from mental hospitals. As he explained to an American interrogation officer after the war, he approached the officials in charge of euthanasia, saying:

> Look here, now, boys, if you are going to kill all these people at least take the brains out, so that the material can be utilized. They asked me: "how many can you examine?" and so I told them an unlimited number. . . . the

more the better. I gave them fixatives, jars and boxes, and instructions
for removing and fixing the brains and they came bringing them like the
delivery van from the furniture company. . . . There was wonderful material among those brains, beautiful mental defectives, malformations and
early infantile diseases. (Mueller-Hill 1988: 67)

Anthropologists, too, were delighted to be able to build collections representing different populations. Eugen Fischer, a leading anthropologist of
the day, was also at the KWI. He worked closely with physicians there and
in Berlin hospitals as well as with Mengele on anthropological and other
medical experiments at Auschwitz. Before the war, to demonstrate racial
exotica, Fischer had gathered together his own extensive collection of anatomical specimens from Germany's former colonies as well as specimens
from Rudolf Virchow's famous private collection. The problem with collecting specimens from the colonies, however, was that researchers had to wait
until a subject died. Organs, tissues, or limbs (including fingernails, arm
sections with tatoos, noses, ears, and so on) were then dissected or preserved with fixatives on the spot. In the concentration camps and hospitals,
on the other hand, both fixed and fresh specimens could be obtained. Camp
prisoners could be killed by injecting phenol directly into the heart, and then
organs could be immediately removed and dissected. Fischer quickly recognized the value of having readily available supplies of fresh specimens
and began to provide his students with camp rather than colony material.
Dr. Johann Paul Kremer also preferred this accessible and plentiful source
of fresh materials to fixed or preserved material: "Kremer looked upon prisoners as so many rabbits" (Lifton 1986: 294).

Body parts were used to create anatomical displays. Heinrich Himmler
asked SS captain and professor of anatomy August Hirt to collect camp specimens to "acquire tangible scientific research material" that would "represent . . . a repulsive but typical species of subhumanity" (cited in Lifton 1986:
285). Photos were taken immediately before killing a victim to document
head appearance, and measurements of the head and face were made. After execution, the head was preserved and the brain and skull examined
for racial classification and pathological features. Himmler anticipated a type
of museum project similar to what Virchow had built in the nineteenth century, with skull, skeleton, and organ displays.

In and of themselves, such collections of specimens are not new or anomalous. Private and public collections of anatomical and pathological specimens were popular in Germany and throughout Europe, particularly in the late eighteenth and early nineteenth centuries. Even earlier, sixteenth-century preternatural philosophers collected nature's anomalies, instituting *Wunderkammern* (wonder cabinets) in Germany (Daston 1995). What differed in this case, aside from the obvious means by which the specimens were acquired, was the sheer volume and variety of specimens not previously available.

The possibilities for research were tempting, even long after the war and public condemnation of the practices. Until recently, many of these same tissue samples and preserved materials were still being used in German medical schools. Professor Hallervorden continued to collect brains and publish research data long after the war, and his collection still exists at the University of Frankfurt. A number of Holocaust sources of material were discovered in East German medical centers after reunification. Although protesters objected to the lack of respect for victims' bodies, it was not until the early 1990s that universities and institutes were forced to stop using the materials and in some cases bury them in designated sites.

The anatomical collection in Berlin was badly damaged by allied bombing. What remains is used privately for teaching students at the medical school where they are housed. Some specimens—mostly pathology specimens from the nineteenth century—are displayed to limited audiences; but hundreds of others remain stacked on crowded shelves, too precious to throw away, too evocative to display to a public (including physicians) that is already sensitive about using humans as display items. When I visited what remains of the Virchow pathological and anatomical collections in 1994, I asked to see the portion that is no longer open to the public. I was led through a series of locked entryways, the last of which opened onto a long hallway filled with tall display cases of skulls, still arranged by race. Most specimens listed a source, such as New Zealand or Rhodesia, and a date of collection, primarily from the late nineteenth century. Many others, however, had neither of these markers but were identified by race or type of anomaly. I was assured that Holocaust sources had been removed from the collection, but this was done only after protests from Berlin's Jewish community.

The Worth of Bodies from "Lives Not Worthy of Living"

A central feature of Nazism was the use of rational technoscience to engineer a planned society meant to last a thousand years. Key to the economic engine of such a society was self-sufficiency and the efficient use and reuse of available materials. In an ultimate act of rationalization, human beings became one such source of recyclable materials.

The planned extermination of millions of "lives not worthy of living" left the government with the problem of how to kill large numbers of people and dispose of the bodies. Gas chambers and large-capacity incineration ovens became the most efficient means of industrialized killing. Eyeglasses, clothes, jewelry, gold dental fillings, and other valuables were removed from the dead bodies and sold or reused. Some camps were able to earn additional income by selling human remains and even the products of incineration. Just about everything from the body could be used or sold: bones for fertilizer, hair for pillows or bed stuffing. Human fat and ashes were used to make soap, as documented in a recipe from the Anatomical Institute in Danzig dated February 15, 1944. Human remains were even used for decorative items. Skin was used for book covers, lampshades, and other ornamental items, often stenciled with designs. Shrunken heads, the products of various attempts to reproduce methods discovered in the colonies, were sold as curios.

Even the process of disposing of the rest of the waste was productive: burning bodies in large-capacity ovens not only destroyed the evidence of genocide but also heated the camp office buildings. Freshly killed bodies burned at a better rate, but cadavers kept in the *Leichenhalle* (storage spaces that held three to four hundred bodies) provided a constant supply.

Thus, humans viewed as refuse could be turned into useful resources for the good of the Reich. Living bodies could provide labor and serve as subjects for experiments to expand medical knowledge. Materials from dead bodies could be used for research, teaching, and commercial purposes. Nothing was wasted; even the products of the remains were used efficiently.

This utilitarian view of human bodies was consistent with Nazi economic policy, which, particularly after 1936, aimed toward greater independence from the world economy. That goal was to be achieved by technological innovation, alternative financing sources, and engineering efficiency, particularly in energy and transportation. Jeffrey Herf (1984) calls this odd coupling of technical and economic rationality with Völkisch nationalist ideology "reactionary modernism." The antimodernist, anticapitalist romanticism of Völkisch thinking in the years leading up to National Socialism were reconciled with modern technology and economic rationality when it became clear that the latter were means to Nazi ideological ends. According to the rhetoric of political romantics, the cultural ideal of "nation" would be reached through the purifying processes of death and violence (Mosse 1964/1981). Thus, military and industrial necessities were transformed into national virtues.

Dealing with the Nazi Past

Revelation of the Nazi atrocities shocked medical communities around the world and brought issues of ethical treatment of patients to the surface. At the Nuremburg trials after the war, physicians on trial for performing human experiments argued that any ethics issues must be judged by German standards alone. During subsequent deliberations and in the writing of the Nuremburg Code, on which modern medical ethics is based, participants adopted many principles from the Reich Health Council Circular of 1931, in spite of the fact that many of these points were ignored in practice during the war—for example, the principle that human experiments should only proceed after animal trials.

The authors of the code based their opinion on the Hippocratic Oath rather than reflecting on the problems of experimentation itself. In other words, the text of the code focuses primarily on how to deal with patients rather than addressing the issue of experimental subjects directly. There is no discussion of informed consent. Benefits to patients, the code suggests, should be balanced against benefits to society at large. This balance continues to be a source of controversy.[7]

The misuse of human bodies under National Socialism has had a profound impact on medical practice, research, and therapy in Germany since the war. The personhood laws in the Basic Law written at the war's end institutionalized a formal concept of human dignity and the protection of the bodily integrity of the living and the dead. This has had direct implications for practice. Today, when any tissue is removed from cadavers, even in the morgue, a number of local and regional regulations apply to the handling of the tissue. For example, an arm amputated in surgery or in an accident must be incinerated intact; no parts of it can be removed for testing or other uses. Parts that are large enough to be recognizable must be incinerated, although other tissue bits can be disposed of with the regular biohazardous waste (f.n., March, August 1994). One pathologist I interviewed felt that having to treat body parts as though they had personhood was ridiculous and interfered with his work: "Even to do biomechanical studies we have to ask permission of the family and of the local ethics committee! Putting the protection of personhood in the foreground really hinders the general good. What if we need more information for a murder investigation?" (f.n., May 1994).

When I asked about the influence of past practices on medical practice today, most physicians said that past practices have nothing to do with contemporary problems associated with acquiring human materials for research or therapy. In fact, no one voluntarily mentioned Nazi medicine in his initial discussion of why procuring and using human materials is more difficult in Germany than in other countries. Some physicians regretted the history of human experimentation and subsequent restrictions on experiments because they would never today be able to do the kinds of investigations necessary to prove certain key physiological principles. For example, the precise moment of death and quantification of damage necessary for death could never be measured (f.n., May, July, August, and September 1994). "We only have extremes here," one physician joked, referring to the extremity of experimentation during the Nazi era and the tight restrictions on any type of human research today.

When pressed, many physicians admitted that past events had affected the public's trust of medicine in general. Public perceptions extend to international scrutiny: many physicians stated a need to act cautiously, not because of changed beliefs or moral compunction but because "the whole world is watching." This partly explains why medical professionals almost never publicly promote organ and tissue donation, nor has there been an organized effort to rebut critics' concerns. Most respondents felt such actions would create even more public discussion of issues that are already sensitive.

Still, not one physician whom I asked said he knew any details of the experiments carried out in the camps. They knew "horrible things were done to people" but were never taught the specifics nor the "logic" behind the experiments—even in medical school, where students are required to take medical history courses. Most of the people who were not physicians said they did not know about medical experiments at all or had only vaguely heard about them.

A handful of respondents were physicians in their mid- to late seventies and would have been in medical school or early in practice during the war. Since many physicians were National Socialists, it is likely that some participated in the human experiments on camp interns or their materials.[8] These physicians avoided answering questions about the effects of the past, focusing instead on improvements in clinical capabilities. They waved away my questions with a uniform response: that's all too far in the past.

One transplant coordinator in his mid-twenties typified comments from younger respondents. He said that Germans should not get stuck in the past; they should build a present and a future they can be proud of. He described growing up watching World War II films from United States, which show Germans as shadowy bad guys. To him, the absence of a strong German identity is like the faceless actor in a military uniform who is never portrayed as a person. In his opinion, it is time to move on. There has been enough repayment and guilt. After all, Germans are now two or three generations away from the perpetrators, and there are more urgent internal and global matters for us to attend to. The past shouldn't make a difference anymore.

As I have shown, there are reasons why the use of the dead for the benefit of the living raises public concern. Since World War II, it has been anathema to speak of community or social body or to suggest that individuals should be selected in some way for the good of the greater society. Ironically, these are precisely the core issues involved in taking human materials from one person for use in another. In the United States, organ transplantation organizations have popularized the motto "donate your organs so that others might live." That motto, however, has a completely different meaning in postwar Germany. Likewise, the consequentialist view—that the dead body is nothing more than organic waste that would otherwise be thrown away—becomes difficult to generalize in the German context.

Coming to terms with the past is an ongoing, everyday activity for Germans. *Vergangenheitsbewältigung,* the process of attempting to manage the past, is something that every activist opposing brain death, every politician, every physician, every citizen must do.[9] Almost all, however, attempt in various ways to distance their work and their everyday lives from the past. Some do this by becoming hypervigilant about potential abuses, while others try to reimagine the past or relegate it to the dustbin of history. Ironically, the language of Nazi violence has been incorporated into contemporary political discourse and often into casual speech (Linke 1995b). In light of efforts to combat images of the past, it is all the more shocking when Nazi themes persist or are trivialized in jokes and popular culture. One egregious example is a video game in which players must establish their racial purity and sell body products and camp labor to earn enough money to exterminate the Turks (*New York Times* 1991).

While changes in the Basic Law, codes of ethical conduct, and medical regulations attempt to isolate and contain the experiences of National Socialism, they are little more than quarantine measures. The work of distancing medical practice from its old identity and creating a new one goes on through formal changes in organization and informal but careful management of work practices. But the nets carefully placed to contain the past require constant maintenance as social changes and new technologies force familiar issues to the surface.

Four

Culture, Technology, and the Law Define the Body

During National Socialism, modernist technology and antimodernist ideology combined to transform persons into things in an extraordinarily efficient manner. The engine of this machine was the particular connection between rational science and romanticist, Völkisch politics and culture. This was a new way of managing society that galvanized Germans into action: individuals were willing to change lifestyles and behaviors, alter family and community structures, follow new moral codes, and make tremendous sacrifices to achieve a unified social body. At the same time, the new rules made it possible to distinguish differences in the worth of individuals using the science of the day. The result was a moral and economic order in which certain persons were designated superior beings encouraged to pursue their true Teutonic path, while others were labeled social refuse.

The bodies of individuals were also differentiated—as either sacred bearer of the German bloodline, contaminating or useless waste, or useful resource. Contemporary societies continue to create such distinctions through our treatment of persons and bodies, living and dead, and the means by which we allow access to certain bodies and their parts. The interpretations we choose become the fulcrum for balancing rights to use and profit from bodily substances. Similarly, the way in which societies handle the dead says much about the treatment of the living.

Changes in German law after World War II formalized the importance of protecting *Menschenwürde* (human dignity and worth). They established the basis for subsequent rules and taboos regarding the body, much of which was directed toward keeping science, technology, and medicine in check. But technological and legal innovations, along with changing attitudes, once again destabilized rules that were meant to guard the dignity of the body and define the boundaries between living and dead. I refer in particular to artificial support technologies and the new diagnosis of brain death, which complicated professional and lay understandings of various states of animation. The technological capability to suspend such in-between states, as well as social and economic pressures to develop life-extending technologies, further challenged notions about proper care and respect for the dead and appropriate uses of bodily remains. In the case of organ transplantation, these new conditions resurrect the question of the social good as opposed to protection and rights of individuals.

Constituting the Postwar German: The Basic Law and Protection of Persons

In the aftermath of World War II, the German social body was eviscerated so that it could never reassemble in quite the same way. Under allied supervision, lands were partitioned, institutions and central governing bodies disbanded, and laws rewritten. New laws explicitly repudiated the treatment of human beings under National Socialism. The *Grundgesetz* (Basic Law), written in 1949, institutionalizes the values of protecting personhood, physical well-being, and individual dignity in its first two articles, known as the *Persönlichkeitsrechte* (personhood rights):

Article I: Human worth, binding nature of the basic law of the state authority

(1) The worth of persons is inviolable. It is the duty of all governmental authority to respect and protect this.

(2) The German people recognize inviolable and inalienable human rights as the basis of peace and justice in the world for every human community.

(3) The following basic rights commit the legislature to the full extent of authority and jurisdiction as the direct valid law.

Article II: Freedom of action; freedom of the person

(1) Everyone has the right to the free expression of his personage as long as he does not injure the rights of another and does nothing against the constitutional order or moral code.

(2) Everyone has the right to life and bodily integrity. Intervention in this right can only be made on grounds of another law.[1]

The principle of *Pietätsempfinden* (a sense of reverence) lies at the heart of these declarations. The laws have been interpreted in subsequent legal codes in very strict ways. The most important of the laws relating to the protection of bodies is paragraph 168 of the *Strafgesetz* (penal code), which refers to *Störung der Totenruhe* (disturbing the dead). The law states that whoever takes or does mischief to a corpse, its ashes, or parts of the body, including those of a dead fetus, or whoever damages or destroys a burial site will be punished by up to three years' imprisonment or pay a fine. In fact, the penalty for disturbing human remains is stronger than the penalty for damaging living bodies—for example, through rape. Even the dignity of burial rituals is protected: paragraph 304 specifies the protection of grave markers, and paragraph 167 punishes the disturbance of funerals with fines or imprisonment.

In its distinctive postwar form, the Basic Law is based on values rather than rights, unlike the U.S. Constitution.[2] The essential concept is the integration of society around a common core of shared values, optimizing competing rights and values to the extent possible in light of universal principles.[3] German courts have read into the Basic Law an objective and hierarchical order of values, topped by the principle of human dignity as stated in the first two articles. Donald Kommers (1995: 18) explains these attempts to combine rights and values: "Each guaranteed right in the Basic Law represents a corresponding value . . . and may obligate the state to create the conditions necessary for the effective exercise of the right. These values are thus a part of the general legal order, constituting an objective morality that social and political reality must mirror." In some situations, then, there may be conflict between rights and values in which values supersede rights. Handling such conflict becomes difficult when trying to balance, for example, the principle of free speech and free press with public protection, as in banning neo-Nazi political activities and publications.

Abortion rulings are another example of the German interpretation of the conflict between rights and values in medicine. The 1975 law that decriminalized abortion was immediately overruled by the argument that the fetus's life, protected by article II (2) of the Basic Law, preempted a woman's right to personal self-determination (found in article II [1]) and that the state is obligated to protect fetal life. The court said that both rights must be determined under the superordinate value of human dignity as stated in article I (1). At reunification in 1990, the law faced another problem because women in the GDR had the right to legal abortions. A new statute was written in 1993 legalizing abortion but supporting social systems that would encourage women to bring pregnancies to term. Ten months later, this law was struck down when, again, the value of protection of life was interpreted to supersede the individual's right to determination.[4] Values can thus be imposed by the state and can be used against the individual if necessary to maintain the state's duty to protect and respect life.

The Basic Law was intended to balance the extremes of individualism and collectivism. Still, abortion, asylum and citizenship, property rights, economic development, and almost all matters in political and public life are decided based on Basic Law values, with articles I and II as master values.

The values feature of German constitutional law is important in understanding the context of attempts to regulate the acquisition and use of human materials. At the time of my research, there was no law to regulate the procurement of materials in Germany other than random local rulings and professional guidelines. But the influence of the Persönlichkeitsrecht is apparent in a code written into the German transplant organization's guidelines: "Protection of the dignity of the dead: The dignity of the dead is to be protected with every measure taken in the removal of organs. The cadaver is to be handled respectfully. The physician is responsible for restoring the outward appearance of the cadaver" (Arbeitsgemeinschaft der Transplantationszentren 1986: 1).

It is interesting to note that the German word for the cadaver's appearance is *Wiederherstellung,* meaning "restoration or restitution" (an act of returning something to its owner and compensating for damage.) In medical usage, the word means "recovery." There is, of course, in organ procurement no recovery or restoration of the body or the appearance to its former state. Nevertheless, it is important to protect the semblance of bodily integrity.

The Persönlichkeitsrechte and their progeny of penal codes and local regulations became the cornerstone upon which a new understanding of personhood and bodily inviolability was built. In that sense, laws became another form of Wiederherstellung. The German body would be restored, but it was the individual autonomous body that would be granted protection, not the society as a collective body. No longer would individuals' bodies be used or disposed of for the good of society because Germans could no longer speak of German society or nation. The laws would be an explicit act of distancing German society from the past.

The terms *pietätsvoll* and *saubervoll* (dignified or respectful), used in the Basic Law to describe how the body should be handled after death, are often repeated in general journalism and medical articles about organ donation. Such language, along with prescribed ways of handling and disposing of the dead, presumes personhood. With the introduction of a number of new technologies, however, various intermediate and ambiguous states of being have been created that call for redefinition.

A Lexicon of the Body

Before discussing the technologies themselves, I wish to introduce the reader to some German terminology. Various states of animation are distinguished linguistically in German using terms that express concepts of the body. *Der Leib* means "the body" and connotes a life essence. It is used in phrases such as *Leib und Seele* (body and soul) but can also refer to the abdomen or gut, a central part of the living body. *Der Körper* also means "the body" but has more to do with the physique and tangible, material corporeality.[5]

Dead human bodies, on the other hand, are called *die Leiche* and *der Leichnam*, both meaning "corpse" or "cadaver"; *die Toten* (the dead, this time without a body); or *die Hirntoten* (the brain dead). *Der Kadaver*, on the other hand, means "carcass" or "dead body," not "cadaver." It usually refers to an animal, although it sometimes appears in pathology texts. Leiche or Leichnam is most commonly used in medical literature, especially to describe the freshly dead or those to be autopsied. The respondents in my study referred to bodies of brain-dead donors of organs and tissues as die Leiche or die Hirntoten during a procurement rather than Körper or Leib. Rarely did I hear an organ donor called "the patient" or "the donor," common terminology in English that connotes the role rather than state of animation. Among medical professionals, body parts are always referred to by specific names: *Hornhaut* (cornea), *Knochen* (bone), and so forth. The terms *sterbliche Überreste* (mortal remains) or *Restkörper* (remains of the body) appear in legal documents or in forensic pathology rather than in general medical writing.

Interestingly, I noted that media accounts of brain death often used Leib interchangeably with Leiche, particularly during the well-publicized case of a pregnant brain-dead woman, which I discuss in chapter 5.[6] The woman's body was referred to as *Mutterleib* or *der Mutter's Leib* (the mother's body), emphasizing her relationship to the fetus; rarely as Leiche; and never as *Frau* (woman). Opposition groups and the media also refer to *Körperteile* (body parts) rather than to specific names of parts.

In short, with the introduction of certain resuscitation and life-extending technologies, *live, dead,* and even *human* have become relative terms. Assumptions of degrees of liveness and humanness are incorporated into contemporary medical-legal classifications of humans and human material. For example, in classifying fetuses and fetal tissue, regardless if they have been born or aborted, categories are based on weight rather than life signs, age, ability to survive, or other characteristics. Until recently, dead newborns weighing less than one thousand grams were classed as *Fehlgeburten* (miscarriages), even if they died after birth. Fetuses weighing up to five hundred grams were registered as *Abort-material* (abortions), not as fetuses. In essence, this meant that a child who survived was counted as a *Mitmenschen* (fellow human being), but one the same weight who did not survive was aborted tissue that was never registered as a person.

Because infants weighing less than one thousand grams survive more often now than they did in the past, the law has recently been modified, indicating the changing boundaries of personhood, life, and death over time. Now nonsurviving fetuses up to five hundred grams remain in the Abort-material category, but those weighing between five hundred and one thousand grams will be counted as *totgeborene Leibesfrüchte* (stillborn) (*Deutsches Ärzteblatt* 1994). This means they will now be registered as persons and can be buried rather than disposed of like other waste tissue, which is usually incinerated in the same way as biohazardous waste.

The ability to detect the cessation of certain brain functions has also shifted the line between what has previously been defined as life and death. Resuscitative technologies developed by the middle of the twentieth century enabled bodies to continue functioning long after the brain had ceased to control these functions, either due to traumatic injury, blockage of blood circulation in the brain, or other brain tissue injury. In 1968 an ad hoc committee created at Harvard Medical School attempted to clarify this new state of being. The Uniform Determination of Death Act, passed by the U.S. Congress in 1981, specified the clinical criteria used to determine when someone was brain dead. Similar definitions and criteria have been accepted in many countries as clear-cut legal and medical designations of death.[7]

As currently defined, brain death is the irreversible and permanent cessation of functions in the whole brain—that is, brain stem functions that control respiration, hunger, thirst, and so on; and upper brain functions that control cognition and awareness, temperature and fluid control, and other regulatory functions. Challenges to this definition stem from the assertion that functions are irreversible and permanent: some detractors argue that it is not known whether function may return at some future time. Moreover, how should one treat cognitive functions? If someone simply has no awareness of her surroundings or ability to interact (common in vegetative states in which brain stem function remains), should she be allowed to die? Or as others have argued, is the loss of what is meaningful in life enough to say that someone has died? These unanswerable questions make it impossible to reach a general consensus on what constitutes death in a technological age. At their base is an assumption that some "real" point of death can be discovered if only there were an ethical way to conduct appropriate tests.

Instead, with the technological capability to sustain a brain-death state, the body sends mixed signals. The usual signs of death—cessation of breathing and heartbeat, a change in color and temperature, among other things—are absent. Instead, with air forced into the lungs by a mechanical ventilator, the body appears to breathe. The skin is a normal color and warm. The body may move: with spinal reflexes, arms and legs can raise and eyelids open (Wetzel, Setzer, Stiff, and Rogers 1985; Ropper 1984). The body appears to be alive. Biological and technological cues, then, must be created: an electroencephalogram printout, representations from imaging technology indicating that certain parts of the brain are blocked from blood circulation, and clinical signs such as fixed and dilated pupils and an absence of breathing reflex now designate when a person is dead. Thus, the patient is marked by signs that he is "dead," but he has not "died." Rather than making the boundaries between life and death more distinct, the new construction of death has left us with an even more ambiguous entity: the living cadaver (Hogle 1995c, Meran and Poliwada 1994, Striebel and Link 1993).

Because of artificial breathing and metabolic support, the death process can be suspended, extended, and staged. It may appear that technology can triumph over nature as mechanical control takes over natural biological and social processes. Yet this liminal state can only exist within the technological milieu of the intensive care unit. The situation is possible only in an era with both the technological capability as well as the social space for a biological body to continue to exist. In this victory of biomedical rationality and the ability to intervene in the dying process, Robert Veatch (1988) poses the question of whether death is a biological fact, a technical construct, or a judgment of legal or theological elites.

Physicians and philosophers who take a biological stance claim that the integration of brain and body functions designate life; they understand the human being as an organism first. Others understand the human as a person first and believe that the conditions for existence, including the ability to interact in the world and integrate into the environment, are determining factors of life. Some have suggested that if we equate the death of the brain to the death of the person, we are saying that the person was only a brain and that the body was nothing more than a vehicle for experience. Here we return to concerns about identity and its connection to organic material, as discussed in chapter 2.

Hans Jonas (1974: 139) suggests that the "extracerebral body" shares identity with the brain: "The body is as uniquely the body of this brain and no other, as the brain is uniquely the brain of this body and no other. . . . My identity is the identity of the whole organism, even if the higher functions of personhood are seated in the brain. . . . Therefore the body—even with the help of art . . . must still be considered a residual continuance of the subject."

These concerns, which have not been satisfied since the first conceptions of the individual, were complicated in western civilizations by early Christianity's tortured definitions of material continuity. In Germany, however, questions of the sanctity of the individual take on heightened significance. The history of euthanasia in Nazi Germany reminds us that the value of particular human lives can be calculated by sentience and by physical, genetic, and mental traits and that these can be malleable elements in determining medical and political policy. This malleability enabled euthanasia programs to expand from passively allowing children with mental illness and other disorders to die to murdering enormous numbers of people who were believed to have no value to society. Claiming that a brain-dead human is no longer a person risks the possibility that too many liberties will be taken. It is the fear of this possibility that makes the concept of brain death and the use of human materials particularly explosive subjects in Germany (cf. *Die Woche* 1994b, Thomas 1993, Wieseman 1995).

The Use of Human Bodies and the Public Good:
The Proposed Transplant Law

By the time the legal designation of brain death was institutionalized in many countries, the removal of kidneys from living donors and transplantation into patients had been going on for some years. Other organs were not possible to transplant because they would cause the donor's death. Researchers had done some experimentation using cadaver organs, but deterioration begins very quickly after the heart stops circulating blood, oxygen, and nutrients through a body. The advent of artificial support technology, combined with the legal definition of brain death, meant that removing and reusing organs from cadavers became possible. Liver, heart, and later lungs and pancreas could be kept functioning within the body of the donor until a recipient was prepared to receive them. Removing the vital organs would not kill the donor because she was already dead, and the organs would not have to be removed after the usual decay had begun.

After a rocky start with poor outcomes in transplant patients, additional technologies were introduced that dramatically improved recipient survival. By the 1980s, the procurement of organs and tissues for transplantation gained the popular image as the power of medical technology to master the failures of nature. Yet the technical ability to collect, preserve, replace, and profit from human materials would have failed without the transformation of cultural ideas about the integrity of the body and its treatment at death. In practical terms, the burial of whole persons had to be seen as a "shameful waste of resources" (Fletcher 1969 :1).

Such changes are not without controversy. In Germany, debates about brain death and the use of human materials occurred while a law to boost organ donation and regulate transplantation services was being debated. Media coverage about organ donation and the proposed law was overwhelmingly negative, focusing on the use of the dead in service to the living, the borderlands of life and death, and the right to self-determination. In contrast, U.S. media coverage focused on the experience of the recipient and the miracle of technology. The only criticisms were directed at the high costs of transplantation or the injustice in allocating scarce organs.

Many new technologies were dubbed invasive because of the ways in which they transgressed boundaries between human bodies and mechanical devices. Indeed, the bodies could not function without the technology, but the technology could not exist without bodies in certain states. In an age of transgressed boundaries, the status of the material body in relation to technology called for new ways of managing the ambiguities that ensued.

In Germany, the absence of clear and consistent laws regarding the procurement and use of human material reflected the uncertainty about the nature of the body, confusion about what constitutes the reverent treatment of the body at death, and questions about the relation of the state to individual bodies. The personhood laws were intended to protect human dignity as the basis of society and guarantee the right to life and bodily integrity. To what extent does this principle hold for the dead also? Discussion about regulating the use and exchange of tissue removed from the body also raised issues concerning the property-like status of cadaver materials. These questions could not be decided by scientific reasoning or moral codes alone. Instead, this medical issue became intertwined in local and national politics and a key theme in debates about society.

At the time of my research, Germany was one of the few countries with no law regarding the procurement and use of organs and tissues for transplantation. Other countries have laws or policies stating either that consent must be obtained from the deceased during his lifetime or from family members at the time of death, or that formal consent is not necessary unless a person objects during his lifetime or if the family objects within a set time, usually a few hours after death. The latter option is known as presumed consent (see table 4.1).

It is important to note that the former East Germany operated under very

_____ Table 4.1 _____
Donation Laws in European Countries, 1996

Law	Countries
Presumed consent	Austria, Finland, Norway, Portugal
Presumed consent but not practiced	Greece, Italy, Spain, Belgium
Informed consent	Denmark, France, Sweden, Switzerland, United Kingdom
No law at time of study	Germany, the Netherlands (presumed consent law in approval process)

Source: Land and Cohen (1992).

different rules. It had laws governing medical procedures for autopsies and for removing organs and tissues for transplantation or research. The latter, called the *Widerspruchslösung,* allowed bodies to be used at the discretion of physicians without permission from family members. According to that law, transplant medicine is a result of scientific progress that promotes and restores the health of citizens; therefore, it allowed the use of organs from the dead unless the deceased had formally registered a contradiction during her lifetime.[8] The laws regarding tissue removal were virtually unknown among the public, and a number of respondents who worked in hospitals in the former GDR told me that families were rarely informed of what happened to their loved ones' bodies after death. At reunification, these laws were abandoned, leaving physicians unsure about how to proceed.

This point about consent is key to the continuing debate in West Germany. The first attempt to pass a national transplant law failed in 1979. The Christian Democratic party (CDU) wanted to have the express consent of the donor, whereas the Social Democrats (SPD) favored presumed consent. There was no consensus on the form and contents, and the draft law was dropped. By the mid-1980s, when it appeared there would be no law, the professional association for transplant medicine substituted a formal statement of guidelines and practice. The advisory committee that drafted the statement consisted of transplant surgeons, a lawyer who has since been active in writing models of presumed consent laws, and representatives of

Protestant and Catholic churches who supported transplantation as an act of Christian charity and a way to save lives.

During my first visit to Germany in late 1992, many physicians told me they were against having a law. They were concerned that it might restrict their practices, believed that it was unnecessary, and thought it brought transplant medicine too much into the public view, where it would be discussed by uninformed people. People not associated with transplant medicine felt that the issues surrounding transplantation paled in comparison with other, more pressing social issues and problems of reunification. This situation changed radically by the end of 1993, when most surgeons I spoke with would have agreed with the respondent who said, "We need a law— any law—we just have to do something about the shortage, get all the bad press over with, and get on with things" (f.n., September 1992). This time, everyone with whom I spoke knew something about the issues involved in the legal battles and expressed concern about the implications.

Health, education, and welfare have all been governed by individual states since the war.[9] In November 1992, at a meeting of health ministers from each state, a new draft of the transplantation law was proposed, this one a type of presumed consent. The health departments of each state had to pass and agree on the exact form before presenting the final draft to the federal parliament. To enact this law would require a constitutional change, placing authority for its execution at the federal rather than the state level. A supplementary paragraph in the federal penal code was also proposed to inhibit and punish anyone trying to sell organs and tissues. But there was no consensus, and politicians became wary as media coverage of the issues stirred public debate. One problem involved state to state discrepancies: the law meant, for example, that tourists going to the wine country could die in an auto accident and have their organs explanted without permission. If a tourist was from Hamburg and had no need to declare his intentions, there would be no registered contradiction.

Meanwhile, two predominant models had been developed. According to *Zustimmungslösung* (the agreement model), the deceased should register her wishes, but relatives must still give permission for doctors to remove organs. In contrast, the *Informationslösung* (the information model, a type of presumed consent law) stated that if the deceased had agreed to donation during his lifetime, organs could be explanted. If he registered a contradiction indicating he did not wish to donate, organs could not be explanted. If there was no information regarding his wishes, then relatives would be informed that organs would be removed. The relatives would have a limited time (four hours in one draft) to contradict the action. If no relatives were found, the coroner could act as a substitute for relatives. Key to this plan was the creation of a central registry to contain each citizen's personal and medical information as well as her intentions regarding the use of her body at death.

Proponents argued that the information model would guarantee many more organs than the agreement model, which more or less codified existing West German practice. The Kuratorium für Dialyse (the national organization that manages dialysis clinics and thus has a financial interest) favored the information model, as did many transplant surgeons and dialysis patient interest groups. That model, however, was hauntingly similar to the GDR's Widerspruchslösung—too close for comfort for many people.

The state of Rheinland-Pfalz went ahead alone and drafted a law at the end of June 1994. Rudolf Scharping, head of the SPD and chief minister of Rheinland-Pfalz, signed a type of presumed consent law that required individuals to register with a central authority and give written notice about disagreeing with donation to avoid being used as a donor. Criticism erupted from all sides, and final passage was delayed.

What happened next is a good example of the kind of collisions that can result when political interests, history, technology, and cultural beliefs meet. Scharping was the SPD candidate in upcoming elections for chancellor. Competing political parties quickly appropriated the topic of organ donation as a way of attacking him personally while clarifying their own positions regarding the relationship between the individual and the state. Representatives from the Green party called Scharping's proposal an *Organbeschaffungsgesetz* (a derogatory label denoting a law that promotes agressive acquisition of organs) and claimed that it was unconstitutional. One CDU parliamentary member called it an "insult against human value" (*Der Spiegel* 1994c: 38). A CDU member of the Rheinland-Pfalz health ministry compared it to the former East Germany's Widerspruchslösung, "the worst thing that could be done to the dead" (38). These attacks focused on the right of the state to claim the bodies of the dead and to make decisions without the express consent of individuals, implying a connection to the past Fascist state.

The uproar bolstered the conservative CDU's portrayal of SPD beliefs as dangerously close to Socialist ideology.[10]

Although national transplant organizations and others supported the law, some supporters of organ donation reversed themselves. Bishop Karl Lehmann, co-author of the transplant association's guidelines and leader of the German Bishops Council, had defended Scharping early on but later urged him not to sign the law (*Ärtze Zeitung* 1994). The debacle was a political disaster for Scharping, who was forced to back down and delay final passage of the law.

Among the law's most vehement opponents was Horst Seehofer, German health minister and member of the conservative Christian Social Union (CSU). He called it a step backward in self-determination for the German people and claimed that it was carelessly thrown together. According to Seehofer, "Er hat uns unheimlich viel Porzellan zerschlagen" (*Frankfurter Allgemeine Zeitung* 1994c). In other words, he believed that Scharping had destroyed the delicate trust in medicine that had been rebuilt after the war.

Seehofer himself had been a direct target in the aftermath of several health care scandals during the early 1990s, particularly one involving HIV-contaminated blood supplies from commercial sources. He was accused of not being able to control the health care system. To counter these attacks, he began projecting an image of himself as both a promulgator of science and a guardian of the overall social good. Organ donation, he declared, is an act of Christian kindness and charity that should not be damaged by dishonoring the dead. But it quickly became apparent that Seehofer's objections were not based on political differences or moral outrage alone. He framed it thus:

> According to Scharping's model, an organ has, in effect, no more protection. Then we have a disastrous situation, when data on [the donor's] identification card are more strongly protected than the organ is. That means that if a physician wanted to diagnose a blood sample for AIDS, he can't do this without express permission. (quoted in *Frankfurter Allgemeine Zeitung* 1994b)

The struggle, then, was as much over control of information about individuals' bodies as over the physical body itself. If there were a central registry in which citizens could exercise their legal right to resist medical intervention, surely this would have implications for collecting tissue, blood samples, or other medical data. Since the abuses of World War II, many people strenuously object to the idea of collecting and centralizing information about individuals as a way of tracking populations and groups. Consider, for example, the number of Germans who refuse to comply with census and epidemiology activities. Scharping's model involved changes in the way in which personal data were recorded and who would have access to them—a source of bitterness in ongoing battles about health care reform among the state, medical care providers, and insurers.

On August 12, 1994, Seehofer and Horst Vilmar, the head of the German Medical Association, announced that Germany should indeed have a transplant law but that self-determination and attention to the right of personhood should be the basis. They endorsed the Zustimmungslösung, including an addendum to punish commercialization activities. Seehofer and Vilmar urged that the transplant law should not be part of the national election debates. They felt Germany was not ready for the type of consensus building this would require since the law would need changes at the constitutional level (*Frankfurter Allgemeine Zeitung* 1994b).

When I analyzed the many proposed versions of the law, I noted that some had additional subtle provisions that have received little public attention. For example, earlier drafts created a central agency in charge of all data handling as well as the organization of procurement and transplantation. Quality control, types of procedures, and data management would be centralized and standardized. Although it was not named in the draft, the Deutsche Stiftung für Organspende (DSO), a German foundation involved in organ donation, lobbied hard for the inclusion of this provision because it assumed the DSO would be in charge of the centralizing process. (See chapters 6 and 7 for more about the DSO.)

Some drafts included a provision for the oversight and regulation of transplant centers, allowing for the possibility of a certification process. To date, there has been little explicit talk of rationing services since that notion connotes "selection," the Nazi term for deciding who would live or be exterminated.[11] Transplant medicine would be the ideal place to begin, especially because it would be the first health issue governed at the federal level.

Effectiveness in transplant medicine is usually tied to experience: therefore, centers with the fewest number of procedures and thus the least experience might be forbidden to continue performing transplants. This has already occurred in Berlin, where there is fierce competition for procedures. At unification, Berlin suddenly had several transplant centers that were now duplicating services. Local authorities have attempted to limit activities of those transplant centers that perform relatively few procedures and prevent them from expanding services to include additional organs.

Further discussions of the law were postponed just before the summer legislative period was over. When I left the country at the end of 1994, they had not been resumed. Since then, debates have continued, centering primarily on how to build consensus among the various states. When I returned in September 1995, the model had changed at least twice, but the presumed consent form was no longer under discussion. Respondents in the transplant field felt this was a disaster: "now the number of refusals will increase to 80 percent!" (f.n., October 1995).

In the most surprising move, the parliament in 1996 considered modifying the definition of brain death, making criteria for diagnosis more stringent. The implication was that organs from bodies not diagnosed according to German rules would be unacceptable. In other words, organs imported from European countries with slightly different criteria could not be used. This political response to the public's doubts about death would have limited the supply even more severely rather than increasing it, as the original draft law intended. In an even more extreme move, the Greens recommended that every individual should define brain death herself, somehow recording that information in a centralized registry.

In 1997 a law was finally passed basically codifying existing practice. That is, procurers will continue to be required to get permission for donation from next of kin.

Cadaver Tissue and Property Rights

At one point there was a move to connect new regulations about autopsies to the new transplantation law, mainly because of the scandals I describe in chapter 5. Medical associations, however, immediately squelched these efforts because they did not want the public to relate the two issues.

For now, dealings with cadavers—autopsy, information needed for determination of death, and disposal of parts—have been left to individual states, while organs from the heart-beating brain dead are regulated at the national level.

When dealing with tissue removed from cadavers in the morgue, the legal principles of protection against *Störung der Totenruhe* (disturbing the dead) and *Körperverletzung* (bodily injury) and the cultural notion of *Pietätsempfinden* (a sense of reverence for the dead) come into play. Whether removed for research, used for data, or processed for therapeutic tools, the basic question comes down to whether the body is a person or a thing and whether the personhood laws even apply.

Practices and regulations are contradictory. Pathologists are required to follow a number of regulations specifically intended to preserve the physical personhood of the body. As I mentioned in chapter 3, an arm amputated in surgery or in an accident must be incinerated intact; no parts can be removed for testing or other uses. Parts large enough to be recognizable must be incinerated, although other tissue bits can be disposed of with the regular biohazardous waste (f.n., March, August 1994). Yet in prevailing legal practice, materials from cadavers are treated as things and endowed with property-like status. For example, one model for a law to regulate materials removed from cadavers claimed that tissue belongs to the state. Pathologists want to control materials themselves and thus object to the law on the grounds that materials can provide important evidence in legal cases.

To whom does the material rightfully belong: the pathologist (or institute), the state, or the individual from whom it came? As one respondent wondered, who is the *Organbesitzer* (who "occupies" the organ or material)? Because the individual's body is no longer human, according to current legal opinion, the individual cannot own anything.

While materials do have characteristics of property once they are removed from the body, commercialization is tacitly prohibited. This prohibition is codified into Austrian law but not German law, at least until the penal code against selling organs comes into effect. Artificial materials in the cadaver, such as pacemakers, are considered to be property foreign to the body. Once implanted, however, they are supposed to be legally removed only with the agreement of the deceased. Making such a declaration does not occur to most of us, so people performing autopsies assume that such devices are treated like cadaver parts, creating another gray area of practice with many controversial results, as chapter 5 will show.

The changes taking place in institutional and organizational arrangements will centralize the state's role in decision making and control. These changes include not only legal definitions but financial structures, including who will pay for which services and procedures. Tied to this issue, of course, is the question of allocation: which and how much of limited goods are given to whom? The power arrangements that develop are central to shaping the nature of evolving German society. What is altruism? What does "the good of society" mean? Both questions show how medical concerns can become enmeshed with broader social issues. Thus, law, customs, and values are as responsible as technological capability and scientific knowledge in shaping how medical science and practice will proceed.

Still, the unresolved cultural questions remain, as journalist Joachim Fritz-Vannahme (1994: 30) shows:

> These [changes] affect deeper-than-religious beliefs in a secular time. Or is this secularization only a thin veneer over archaic ideas, for which a corpse as far as anyone knows is now just an object without a soul? Here, not only rights and interests collide. The worth of the dying, the need of the affected, and the duty of physicians are at stake. Have we left those who perform transplantations alone too long with these decisions? With the right of our own body [at stake], might their justifications just be a defense of the principles of individualistic society? Is it going too far to think of the body as only material? That should be decided by individuals, not by law.

Rights, Values, and Bodily Inviolability

Linda McLain (1995) observes that imagery of bodily inviolability often employs spatial relations to convey a sense of inaccessability. For example, Hans Jonas's (1974) location of personhood and the right of control over one's body begins at the skin. But regardless of how it is perceived, what constitutes a personal violation can be redefined when the use of bodily substances seems to serve purposes justified by supraordinate needs or goals.

There have been a number of precedents in which the state's rights over and access to human bodies are seen to supercede the individual's rights to control and make decisions about his own body. Public health measures such as quarantine and mandated vaccination programs show that individual bodies can be construed as threats to the general well-being of the public, justifying enforcement of state authority. For example, in the United States one man's refusal to receive the smallpox vaccine highlighted the government's authority to violate an individual's body on behalf of public safety (Jacobson v. Massachusetts 197 U.S. 11 [1905]).[12] Drug testing and body searches set civil rights and employer or governmental rights in opposition to each other. HIV-infected persons who knowingly have unprotected sex are subject to punitive statutes controlling their private behavior. In such cases the physical status of an individual body, whether infected or a carrier of contamination or dangerous elements, is perceived as threat to the social order. The threat associated with individuals' bodies must be contained, purified, or removed using external social and technological means. Alternatively, the threat can be defused internally by enhancing the immune system or altering the genes—a new way of managing social hygiene.[13]

In contrast, in procurement and transplantation, it is the shortage of organs and tissues that is portrayed as the threat to the social order. Certain end-stage organ failures are reconceived as a major public need rather than the need of specific people. Framing individuals as the gatekeepers of an important societal resource—their own healthy body parts that could help other people—relies upon certain understandings of altruism and what belongs in the public domain. To suggest that individuals have a *duty* to give up parts of their bodies is based on an idea of protecting the welfare of society as a whole. This enables authorities to discuss even the possibility of a legal right of access to the body parts of citizens.[14]

In Germany, it was remarkable that a presumed consent law was proposed at all, given the mixture of biology and politics that transformed history only a half-century ago. For the concept of entitlement to work, the protection of bodily integrity as it was understood in the postwar constitution would have to be reinterpreted. The private matter of dying and the negotiations between families and medical practitioners would become public and subject to dispute at court and constitutional levels.[15] Entitlement would need to be constructed in ways making it distinctly different from both the wartime atrocities and the GDR's Socialist state authority. The values orientation of the Basic Law would have to be interpreted so that a law enabling access—and enforcing sharing—would be serving the public good. To use biology as a means of moving toward social solidarity would reformulate a ritual of national identity but in a very problematic way. In chapter 5, I examine the thorny issue of sharing and moral community as they mingle with ideas about individual boundaries and state authority.

Five

Bodies, Sciences, and the State in the New Germany

In the late twentieth century, Germans must confront the issue of how to balance the protection of persons as individuals with the increasingly complex needs of society. In the aftermath of reunification and with tens of thousands of immigrants and fierce competition in the international economy, Germany finds itself reconsidering old questions about the social body. What is worth sacrificing for the good of society? What claims over the lives and bodies of societal members can be made on behalf of scientific progress or economic survival? How far should the state or medical science go to protect the dignity of a person when there may be greater gains to be had for a greater number of people, especially if that person is already dead?

The Basic Law, as discussed in chapter 4, was designed to demarcate a boundary between the state and individuals, but its authors could not have foreseen some of the complex dilemmas facing Germany in the late twentieth century. While article II guarantees the protection of persons and the inviolability of their bodies, several events occurred during my fieldwork that forced Germans once again to confront issues of bodily violation. The cases I discuss in this chapter involved using dead bodies for questionable purposes. Most disturbing was the fact that these were not single incidents but revelations of routine practices. Thus, many people saw them as emblematic of the invisible machinations of medicine and industry, which were once more operating on the bodies of the people. These events destabilized professional and popular conceptions of death, the proper treatment of the dead, and the appropriate application of medical technology.

The cases provide a glimpse into the interactions among practices, responses to them, and the ways in which both are represented by various sources. Within these interactions, cultural understandings and rules may shift and new conditions be forged in which questions of inviolability, entitlement, and the public good are formulated. It becomes clear that cultural resistance is homogenous in neither content, expression, nor effects.

Constructions of Life and Death: The Erlangen Experiment

Marian Ploch, a young woman from Erlangen, was declared brain dead after sustaining head injuries in a car accident. She was thirteen weeks' pregnant.[1] Her physicians decided to continue to artificially support her body in the attempt to preserve the life of the fetus. There have been other cases of postmortem maternal ventilation, but they involved more fully developed fetuses that could soon be viable on their own. Normally, artificial support can only be extended for a few weeks in a brain-dead body; after that, the body's physiology begins to fail, and too many complications set in. Because life support had never been attempted for such a long time, many critics saw it as a test of the limits of medical technology. Thus, the case came to be known in the media as the Erlangen Experiment.

Public reaction became hostile as details of the case were revealed. Many chemical and mechanical technologies were necessary to sustain the woman's body in its brain-dead state. Artificial nutrition was provided, bringing up questions about whether a cadaver could or should be fed. Hormones were administered to approximate the woman's normal pregnant state. When the kidneys began to fail, the body was mechanically dialyzed. One eye became infected and was removed since antibiotics could not be infused because of the fetus. Her body was moved as if it were exercising, and other activities were planned to provide a "natural" setting for the fetus. Nurses talked to the fetus and played music, saying, "It's happy when it hears beautiful music" (*Der Spiegel* 1992: 324). In short, medical personnel took aggressive measures, but the effort was directed toward keeping a safe environment for the fetus rather than treating the woman either as a patient or as a person who had just died.

Overcoming technical difficulties was only part of the problem. Things became more ambiguous when the coroner refused to sign a death certificate for the woman, saying the fetus would then be born with no mother, which the coroner claimed would be a technical impossibility. The woman, then, was legally but not officially dead. This unleashed a furious exchange in the popular and medical literature. One poll showed that 82 percent of those surveyed thought the woman and the baby should be allowed to die.[2]

In the legal decision to continue the pregnancy, the judge said that no one had the right actively to kill a baby (*Deutsches Ärzteblatt* 1993: 74). The clinic spokesperson, Dr. Franz Gall, framed the issue as the child's right to life, which was guaranteed by the personhood laws. This right mandated the use of all modern technological methods available. But many people saw the situation as a macabre and unnatural treatment of the dead, indicating a lack of Pietätsempfinden as called for by the same constitutional law. The debate concerned the rights of the dead versus the need to protect the living—a values over rights claim. Decisions about the fetus belonged to the woman's parents, but the interests of the woman herself were unclear because there was no law to regulate the care of legally dead people (*Tagespiegel* 1992).[3] After some time, Marion's parents tried to withdraw their consent to the procedures, but attending physicians countered with attempts to remove their rights to custody of their daughter's body.

For years the Harvard brain-death definition had been generally acknowledged as a definition of death acceptable in many countries. This case, however, stimulated concerns about the nature of the dying process. More important, it flagged the issue of the right of medical experts to determine when someone is dead and in whose interest that claim could be made. The original message used to convince the public to accept brain death as a legal determination of death had been that irreversible damage to certain brain functions meant death of the whole person, including the body.[4] Organs and tissues could be used for someone else if they were removed very quickly; otherwise, they were nothing more than dead waste material. Because physicians in this case were claiming that the dead body contained life, the argument became dicier.

Articles written during this time, for both the medical profession and the public, began to use new terminology and descriptions of brain death and the body. They described the "ongoing life" of the body's materials, even though the body as a whole could no longer survive. Language shifted away from terms connoting an entirely dead entity (Angstwurm 1987, 1990; Haupt et al. 1993). Now there was a separation between the brain as a dead organ and organic materials that continued to have generative ability—if they were used quickly and well:

> "Death occurs when the central organizing organ is destroyed, not when cells and tissues stop functioning." (Klein 1995: 9)

> "Death is a process; parts of the body continue to live with appropriate support." (Birnbacher et al. 1993: 2928; see also Meran and Poliwada 1992)

The line that had seemed so clear blurred once again. Not just a live organ but an entire person's life was at stake.

The fetus aborted after six weeks, to the shock of physicians. It was reported to be a natural death: "the child came into the world dead at 00:10" (*Tagespiegel* 1992: 30). Other accounts, however, gave the fetus more direct agency, with these headlines:

> "With the exit of the fetus, Germany's extraordinary experiment is at an end."

> "Fetus ends clinic experiment." (Gast 1992:2)

> "Departure of the Erlanger fetus; dead mother turned off" (*Tageszeitung* 1992: 2)

The phrase "turned off" was problematic, suggesting that the woman's body could be switched on and off like an incubator. After the long ordeal, the family refused to allow autopsies on the fetus or the woman, and local authorities barred physicians from further investigations.

The definitions of life and death employed in this case were contested by a variety of interested actors, including anti-abortion activists, biomedical researchers, and religious groups. The fetus and the woman became variably understood entities: political symbols, cultural icons, experiments, or statements about the moral status of persons. In a sense, the fetus also became an active agent in determining the application of technology. Handled like a fetal container, the brain-dead woman became a battlefield for the combat between the authority of medical practitioners and scientists versus the rights of individual citizens.[5]

By this point, arguments had been extended to the treatment of other brain-dead patients—in particular, potential organ donors. Members of the medical profession were concerned about the articles and editorials criticizing the handling of the case and publicizing growing doubts about brain death (cf. Brautigam 1994, Hoefling 1994, Taupitz 1994). A number of new books were focusing on brain death, especially in connection with organ transplantation. In *Wann ist der Mensch Tot?* (When is a person dead?), Johannes Hoff and Jürgen in der Schmitten (1994) collected medical descriptions as well as debates by philosophers, theologians, and journalists. Other books offered evidence that life continues after brain death or accused medical practitioners of mistreating the dead (Greinert and Wuttke 1993, Striebel and Link 1993).

The well-publicized case of postmortem maternal ventilation threatened the carefully constructed rules for determining the boundaries of death and life. Several years later, the case still evokes strong reactions from the public, medical professionals, and ethicists whom I interviewed. When discussing understandings of death and appropriate treatment of dead bodies, both laypeople and physicians invariably invoked it as a cautionary tale.

Mistrust of Medicine: Donor Ambulances, Human Crash Test Dummies, and the Sale of Cadaver Parts

The normality of the health system is the problem, not the criminal cases.
  (*Der Spiegel* 1994a)

The image of a dead woman's body as an experimental object, manipulated in ways to which she never agreed, evoked memories of Nazi medical experimentation. To many, it became a symbol of the pursuit of scientific and technological progress at the expense of the dignity of the person. But the feeling that German medicine and physicians could not be trusted had already been intensified by other scandals involving shocking uses of humans and their remains. Common to representations of these scandals were ideas about the unanticipated consequences of death and the powerlessness of people to protect the dignity of the dead.

In this section I discuss three cases in particular: a scandal alleging premature organ removal in the former GDR, the use of cadavers as crash test dummies, and the selling of tissue and prostheses from cadavers in hospitals. In each case, the revelation of what appeared to be routine practice awakened the fear that control over the dead was often in the hands of authorities pursuing their own interests.

Donor Ambulances

Not surprisingly, the scandal in the former GDR had a political twist. Patients who were severely brain damaged were often brought into major medical centers to determine if they were brain dead because equipment and specialists were not always available in small-town clinics. In late 1989 a story broke claiming that specially designed ambulances were taking away patients who were not yet dead and bringing them to the Charité, the largest and best-equipped university clinic in East Berlin. There they were diagnosed as brain dead, and organs and tissues were removed (Stein 1992).[6] This was the first that most East Germans in general had heard about the Widerspruchslösung—the law allowing the use of bodies without permission. Western media coverage invoked an atmosphere of horror: allegations grew into suggestions that patients were being snatched from their hospital beds and carried away—perhaps even declared dead prematurely—without the knowledge or permission of families. Some articles even implicated the Stasi (Wuttke 1991). According to the westerners who spoke with me, this was another example of the horrors of state control over individuals' lives and bodies.

The news, however, seems to have had different local meanings. In my discussions with East Germans, I learned that they, too, were furious that procedures were being done without their knowledge. They felt that the practice was little different from the Stasi's surveillance, political arrests, and many other government activities that invaded individuals' privacy and violated human rights. Just as incendiary, however, was the belief that this was another typical example of all money and resources going to Berlin to serve party functionaries and privileged members of society at the expense of the brotherhood of workers: "Berlin got everything—all the money, the best clinics, and public services, and now we learn [that they got] all our organs, too!" (f.n., April 1994).

Procurement and allocation of organs and tissues were centralized in Berlin and theoretically could have been allocated to any East German or to patients in allied Eastern bloc countries that participated in organ exchanges. In practice, however, working-class individuals living in outlying areas, while having access to primary care, had far less access to diagnostic technologies and specialists who could place them on waiting lists for organs.[7] Physicians in my study admitted that higher-ranking party members and key individuals enjoyed a different tier of medical care and coverage.

The central issues concerned control and rights over human bodies. Who has a right to use citizens for which purposes, and who has a duty to care for the dead? The story was exposed just when East Germans were discovering proof about the injustices of their former government. Thus, they received a double shock: individuals and their bodies quite literally belonged to the state and were used to benefit the privileged few.

Human Crash Test Dummies

In the wake of the donor ambulance story, a series of newspaper articles in November 1993 revealed that human cadavers were being used in place of artificial dummies to perform crash tests for auto safety. Effects of the tests on the bodies were described in graphic detail, complete with grotesque photos. Media coverage focused on the physical destruction of the bodies. Stories depicted cold and ruthless experimenters with no respect for people. Headlines such as "What happens to me after my death?" expressed the public's feeling of powerlessness when individuals were up against big industry and science (*Bild-Zeitung* 1993: 1). Interestingly, none of the many media accounts that I collected referred to human experimentation more generally or to the history of the use of human bodies in Germany. In contrast, U.S. accounts of the crash tests explicitly referred to Nazi medical experiments (*San Francisco Chronicle* 1993).[8] Nevertheless, the public was outraged about what it perceived as body mutilation.

The auto safety industry justified the practice, appealing to the need for rational science and progress. Researchers from the Safety Institute at the University of Heidelberg, where the tests were performed, claimed it was necessary to use human bodies to determine if bodily damage sustained in crashes would be deadly or merely injurious. To the horror of fellow scientists, researchers invoked the very example physicians were attempting to soothe public fears about: "With an autopsy or an organ transplant a lifeless body is no less horribly disfigured, and so far no one has urged that we should forbid sectioning a cadaver" (*Der Spiegel* 1993b: 210).

More provocative, however, was the claim that such experimentation was necessary to test the efficacy of the artificial dummies: "Human cadavers give more exact measurements than dummies. Test dummies must be altered to copy humans better" (*Bild-Zeitung* 1993: 2). In this case, human material was used to estimate the accuracy of reproduction in technical products rather than technology used to substitute for human characteristics or skills. The disturbing message was that human remains were used in the service not only of the state but of machines as well.

Just as disturbing as the actual use was the way in which the bodies were acquired. Experimenters could not prove that permission from relatives was granted to use the bodies. There were also charges that some relatives were paid for the bodies, raising the issue of a market for human bodies. This allegation was not proven, but one spokesperson said that there was no wrong done precisely because the materials were paid for.

What made the greatest impact on authorities was the admission that children's bodies were used, breaking a taboo even within the safety industry. After this finding, forensic medicine authorities claimed that the case was, indeed, one of Störung der Totenruhe. The Vatican chastised the individuals involved, and finally the federal government ordered a scrutiny of research practices. As a result, the researchers ceased using children's bodies but continued to use adults'. Again we ask, which kinds of goods—or which humans—have value for what purposes? Which are not to be violated and why? The public admonition from governmental authorities produced a paper image of control and a measure of assurance for the public, but in effect the practice continues almost unchanged.

The Sale of Cadaver Materials

In 1994 the public was shocked once again: by the revelation that materials were being removed from cadavers in hospital morgues and sold to pharmaceutical companies. Pathology workers removed materials such as dura mater, whole brains, pituitary glands, connective tissue, bones of the extremities and the inner ear, and other tissues and gave or sold them either to brokers or directly to pharmaceutical and other firms. This practice had been going on for many years in Germany and other countries, stimulated by the growing demand for human material for research and for processing into other products. Prosthetic devices were also removed and sold to firms that recycled the materials; a jeweler in Kassel paid thirty marks per gram for titanium hip joints (*Der Spiegel* 1993c: 72). Workers averaged between three and five hundred extra marks per month by selling these materials, and occasionally the clinic was also paid.

Although pathologists denied participating, they admitted to looking the other way because pathology workers receive relatively low pay and are difficult to recruit. There was tacit agreement that the practice was in order and that receiving money was compensation for an undesirable job. A pathologist defending the practice told me: "I can't find anything bad about it. Dura mater [taken during autopsy] is just a waste product" (f.n., August 1994). Several clinics justified giving dura mater to firms because there was no artificial substitute: "the brain injured and children with spina bifida can be helped" (*Der Spiegel* 1994b: 143). Another pathologist used a different argument: "If we don't collect this [tissue] here, we will have to get it from Southeast Asia. That's not good. We need to know that it's the same kind of tissue [as tissue in Germany] and that it's clean and safe" (f.n., September 1994). For this pathologist, the possible lack of safety testing for HIV or other infective agents at the collection site was a problem, as was the fact that the tissue itself might have different qualities. He felt that mentioning the threat of potential contamination would make the public see that allowing the collection of tissue at home was more beneficial for potential patients.

Media tactics fueled public outrage. Amid references to "plundering the dead," the media printed stark photographs of piles of bones, heaps of artificial hip joints, and large containers of brains—much like the piles of human hair, skin, bones, eyeglasses, and dental prostheses displayed when the concentration camps were liberated.

Legally and ethically, several issues were at stake. First, hospitals often presumed that permission to carry out the autopsy implied consent to use the materials. Germany has no specific informed consent law regarding the acquisition of materials from the cadaver itself, much less giving or selling materials to other parties. Tissue is not supposed to be removed without express permission, "unless it is needed"—a loophole allowing pathologists to use their own discretion.

Another problem was payment. The media referred to sales of the tissue as *Organhandel*, a word suggesting that all organs and body parts were sold rather than donated. At the time of my research, there was no law forbidding sales of human body parts. Instead, there was a tacit understanding that unused materials could be passed on for research or other use. For many years, German firms such as Braun and Biodynamics acquired tissues (especially pituitary glands from which to extract growth hormone) from the GDR, the Czech Republic, and other eastern European countries, where there was less restriction and less public knowledge or reaction about the practice.

Most controversial was the question of whether the practice disturbed the peace of the dead. Is removing tissue from the body, no matter how small, a disturbance? According to defenders of the practice, as long as the overall body remains intact, there is no problem. As one pathologist said, "If, for example, two hundred grams of tissue were taken for industry, that's only 0.2 percent of a normal person" (*Der Spiegel* 1994b: 142; Ulrich and Geschonneck 1994). To him, such a small amount of tissue did not constitute a violation.

Politicians quickly joined the fray. Representatives of the SPD (a party somewhat oriented to the left) and the Green party spoke out against the practice on the principle that profit should not be made from selling bodily materials. Many politicians, however, defended the use of cadaver material since it could extend or improve the lives of other people. In the end, several workers were suspended from their jobs but were not otherwise penalized, and hospitals were warned "not to be left to the temptation of industry" (Dr. Helmut Becker, representative of the physicians' association in Berlin, February 24, 1994).

Resistance and Reinterpretation: Organized Opposition

Each scandal was accompanied by a barrage of media coverage and became the chief topic of many evening news reports and talk shows. The stories stirred up public sentiment and fueled the fires of various individuals and groups who opposed the use of human bodies for other purposes, including transplant medicine.

Opposition to the use of human materials takes several forms and stems from disparate sources. Perhaps the most organized group is GenArchiv, founded in 1985 to protest genetic engineering. Since then, it has expanded to include a number of health concerns, such as environmental issues and access to care, primarily as they affect women. GenArchiv began to target organ and tissue transplantation in about 1992. Participants are oriented on the political left; several are active in the Green party, and others are active in FINRAGE, a leftist feminist group. A similar but smaller group, the Genetische Network, operates out of Berlin.

GenArchiv members publish broadly, hold workshops, and collect data and articles for distribution. Their goals, however, reach beyond public education. Although they do not hold demonstrations, they do attend pro-donation meetings and challenge speakers. Individuals cite several reasons for participating in GenArchiv, but most center around a general criticism of medicine and the way in which the medicalization of certain social conditions changes peoples' lives. As one person told me, "people in Germany expect physicians to be everything—priest, friend, healer. We need to break patients' blind trust of physicians" (f.n., February 1994). Regarding transplant medicine and the use of cadavers for crash tests, another respondent commented: "Our question is, what sort of science is this that requires bodies for research? This has become normal science—like the normal science of eugenics [under Nazism]" (f.n., February 1994).

When I questioned transplant surgeons and coordinators about GenArchiv, they all knew about the group but considered it more of an irritant than a threat. Clearly, however, the organization is taken seriously in some quarters: in 1987, after a genetics research laboratory was bombed, GenArchiv members became the chief suspects. According to the members I interviewed, offices and homes were raided, with all files removed and many not returned. The women were strip-searched, and two were imprisoned—one for eight months—without evidence.

Other opposition groups have worked to inject Protestant Christian ideas into debates on brain death and transplantation. One such effort, led by theologian Klaus-Peter Jörns, is called the Berliner Initiative. While Jörns does not oppose the practice of transplantation per se, he objects to any law that controls or encourages automatic donation of organs (Jörns 1993). Specifically, he objects to the idea that people are obliged to give their bodies to society. According to the initiative's position statement, which appears on its petition, "Christian belief and psychosomatic medicine understand humans as a body-soul unity, and this must be protected. . . . The body is no shell from which an immortal soul departs, thrown away as having become meaningless in death; rather, it belongs inseparably to the persona of each individual human." The statement goes on to declare that organ donation is not a Christian duty.

Jörns questions whether brain death should be used as a legitimate definition of death. He believes that loss of brain function does not represent the death of the body-soul unity and that to claim so opens the possibility of abuse. He specifically names the Erlanger baby to support his case. He also warns that transplant medicine uses the victims of society, thereby creating an *Über-wir* status (a type of super-collective society), with physicians having power over the poor and oppressed (f.n., May 1994).[9] His word choice recalls *Übermensch,* a National Socialist term for a superhuman race.

Jörns has circulated his position statement and started a petition that had several thousand names, including those of politicians and physicians. He has appeared frequently on television and radio talk shows along with his physician wife, Dr. Wiltrud Kemstock-Jörns.

A number of physicians, clergy, and others oppose various facets of organ and tissue procurement and transplantation, for reasons primarily related to questions about brain death and the autonomy of the individual. Their arguments consider disruption of body integrity, disturbance of personhood both for the dead donor and the recipient of his organs, as well as a too-powerful medical establishment that intervenes in individuals' lives (Ranke-Heineman 1992).

Remembering and Re-membering: Public Good, Public Image, and Private Fears

The transplant physicians and researchers whom I interviewed blamed the media for the current tissue shortages in Germany. They felt that journalists were irresponsible when they reported on scandals, that they just wanted to sell a story. Several thousand items on organ donation, brain death, and transplantation appeared in the German media in 1994, almost all of them unfavorable.[10] Yet critics of the media sidestep the content of most of these accounts, focusing their attacks on media coverage of problems outside Germany. According to one transplant surgeon, "organ transplantation has suffered a strong setback in Germany due to the negative reporting of the media, which denounces abuses—assumed or real—that occur in other cultures and other countries" (Pichlmayer 1991).

It is unlikely that, alone, a generalized mistrust of medicine or fear of bodily destruction (even if stimulated by media stories or urban myths) accounts for Germans' negative perceptions of organ donation. Rather, the scandals have disrupted powerful expectations about the protection of persons, even (perhaps especially) the dead.

The generation that grew up during National Socialism was bombarded by images of strength, vigor, and purity as representations of the true German body. In Nazi sculpture, art, and propaganda people saw a body emblematic of German society. This image of classical perfection became vulnerable only in the presence of degenerate, broken bodies. Jews, homosexuals, criminals, and the disabled were depicted as bent, deformed, infectious, and contaminating.[11] As I have discussed, the body became a political and cultural symbol of nation and society.

In postwar laws, the body persists as a political icon, but now as a recovered body. It demonstrates the repentance of the state and the restitution of pre-Nazi protections. Younger generations did not grow up with the images that bombarded their parents; in fact, they saw few representations of nation or of the collective political body.

The cases I have discussed in this chapter were publicized through graphic images of damaged, vulnerable bodies. Photographs showed naked, ripped cadavers splayed in morgues and wrecked cars, piles of body parts in bins. Just as images of the racially pure Nazi body were not neutral, the cadavers described in these stories were not simply objectified bodies without meaning. Instead, the circulation of stories compelled engagement with the spectacle. By provoking a reaction, the body again became a trenchant symbol of force, but this time there was no single focal source of power.

This symbol, however, can be interpreted in various ways. As Adele Clarke and Theresa Montini (1993) have shown in their discussion of contested technologies, the groups concerned with the use of human materials, as well as the political and economic interests and technologies, have histories themselves. To some, the body and its parts reconfirm religious ideas. Others use bodies as cultural icons. For others, they are commodified or commercializable work objects. Still others use the battle over bodies to reinterpret political commitments. And in subtle ways, the handling of bodily materials becomes, for some people, a way of sustaining the hierarchy of expertise. While each of these arenas may have its own particular history, other layers of history underlie them all—not just the murder and human experimentation under the Nazis but also the violations of bodily privacy under the East German regime. The long and tortured history of Germanic territories struggling to define their relation to each other adds unresolved dimensions of duty and belonging. These layers of old and new ideas can in no way be understood as traditional cultural resistance to late twentieth-century bodily practices.

Nevertheless, narratives of resistance and reinterpretation offer alternative accounts of a contested technology. By working out ideas outside the laboratory or the hospital intensive care unit, they actively construct knowledge. As we saw in chapter 4, such alternative knowledge can interact with and influence policy and affect the choices and attitudes of the individuals directly responsible for collecting materials from bodies.

In a sense, the spectacles of the early 1990s are similar to premodern spectacles of torture and punishment. Here, however, observers react to the representations of what is being done to bodies rather than the direct action itself. Moreover, it is not punishment that is being enacted but the transformation of the body's role in society. In *Discipline and Punish,* Michel Foucault (1979) describes the spectacles as a necessarily public form of punishment. Crimes, he explains, were an affront to the sovereign as the incorporation of the political body. But public reaction was unpredictable; crowds could observe, or they could object, even riot. If they rioted, judgments were made in private, with outcomes determined by judicial or ecclesiastical elites.

In the modern nation-state, the affront is not against the individual king's body as representing governance but against a representation of the collective social body. The government responsible for protecting the collective of individuals has been exposed as allowing—or perhaps enabling—deviances in practice. In the spectacles I have described in this chapter, this revelation of deviance exposed the vulnerability of constitutional protections written specifically to inhibit the state's abuse of power over individuals' bodies—at least symbolically.

It might appear, then, that the media images represented voices of resistance from the people. I suggest instead that through media stories, public responses, and subsequent opposition activities, various points of resistance were allowed to be articulated. That is, the various understandings of human bodies stemmed from a number of different points of resistance to, acceptance of, or accommodation to "spectacular" bodily practices. Some of these understandings were based on religious beliefs, others on political ideology, still others on economics. As voices began to interact, opposition groups found a kernel around which to organize action, industries adjusted investments or public relations campaigns, individuals reevaluated their own beliefs or their relationships with physicians, and politicians crafted party platforms.

In the wake of each of these events, federal and local government authorities researched issues and made various recommendations, but little changed. The practice of using human cadavers for crash tests had been going on for twenty-eight years. Press reports from the 1960s and 1970s stimulated similar protests. Spokespeople at that time defended the practice, saying the tests would lead to better seatbelt designs. The tests continued. The commercial use of cadaver materials has also been going on for a number years; and despite this recent uproar, no law has been passed to strictly forbid it. Although individuals can no longer be paid, institutions can still collect materials and be reimbursed for them.

In the modern nation-state, it is no longer a question of the right of an individual sovereign to violate a person's body. Rather, individuals collectively may permit certain kinds of violation to proceed simply in order to exist in this type of social order. Displays of the order are made public and visible through certain political rituals—dramatizations to create the appearance of control and containment. Public representations of spectacles and the varied responses to them create a space in which these dramatizations can take place. People can raise questions about the inviolability of bodies and persons, thus providing an appearance of democracy. Some technologies and legal and economic arrangements may shift, but the outcomes are left open for interpretation. In part 2 of this book, I show how the form that institutions and organizations take can be shaped by the concerns that alternative knowledge raises.

Part II
Medical Practice and the Politics of Redemption

The value of human materials as healing tools depends not only on their inherent biological functions and attributed symbolic power but societies' ability to garner the resources necessary to acquire the right materials, process them into usable form, and transport them to potential users. Otherwise, tissue would be useless, no matter how advanced the technology for which it was ultimately intended.

To understand fully the practices involved in human materials technology, we must identify all aspects of and participants in the enterprise. Thus far, I have scanned the cultural, political, and historical aspects that affect and are affected by technoscientific endeavors in particular contexts. Such factors play an important role not only in the form that technologies take but in the application of scientific theories that underlie them. Theories about the physiology of maintaining the artificial support of a donor, immunology and tissue matching, and ways of thinking about how to preserve and store human tissue and other technical aspects are, of course, key to understanding practices surrounding human materials use. Yet there are other central, if less visible, elements, including the organizational arrangements for obtaining and processing materials, the means of funding, and regulations and other ways of managing the work. Procedures, skills and techniques, materials and instruments, and the sites where the work occurs all play a significant role in shaping medical work. This idea has become commonplace in the social study of science and technology.[1]

Nevertheless, organ and tissue donation has a very different public face. The common perception of organ procurement is something like this: a person becomes brain dead. The organs and tissues are immediately removed by a team of surgeons in the hospital where the patient has died. The name of a recipient is provided by an impartial computer from an objectively ranked list of candidates. The organs are rushed by helicopter to the recipient, who is the next person on a waiting list; or as some people imagine, organs are walked down the hall to another patient in the same hospital.

In fact, there is a great deal more to the story. The chapters in part 2 let us peer behind these public representations of organ procurement to examine the necessary activities, participants, and structures at transnational, national, and local levels. Arrangements are extraordinarily complex, differing according to type of organ, classification systems of recipients and materials, and variations in regional or local practice. Adherence to supposedly agreed-upon and universal policies based on "medical" and "social" criteria also differs at the local level, further complicating the situation.

It is impossible to tease apart the steps of the process in either a chronological or a macro- to microlevel way. For this reason, I devote the rest of this introduction to a brief overview of the interwoven activities expanded upon in the following chapters, following the organs and tissues as they move from one space to another. Their movement may take the form of information flows, as data that represent human materials course from bedside through modems to network computers. This flow reshapes the proxy tissue as surely as the organic matter itself is processed into usable therapeutic implements.

When a patient has a brain injury that is severe enough that it is unlikely she will survive, a neurologist and at least one other physician follow a clinical protocol to test for brain function. Neither doctor can be associated with transplant medicine. If the tests indicate the cessation of blood flow and irreversible loss of function consistent with the definition of brain death used in that country, the family is notified. The patient is usually already on artificial support and in the intensive care unit. Otherwise, she is moved there, where the body will remain until it is transferred to surgery for organ removal, if the family gives permission.

Most countries have a network organization that facilitates organ procurement and transplantation. The network in the United States is called the United Network for Organ Sharing (UNOS). UNOS contracts with regional organ procurement organizations (OPOs), which are not-for-profit organizations, independent of the hospital-based transplant centers responsible for organ transplantation.

Someone at the hospital will notify the OPO.[2] If the patient seems to be a good candidate for organ donation, a trained professional from the OPO will go to the hospital and immediately begin clinical management, often taking over for hospital staff. This process may begin before brain death is actually diagnosed (Hogle 1993).

A few hours are allowed to pass after the family has been notified of the brain death. Then an OPO representative or sometimes the physician will ask the family for permission to take organs and tissues for transplantation. If permission is granted, the OPO representative continues to provide clinical management along with hospital staff until the time of removal while organizing the logistics of the procedure itself. These clinically trained personnel, called procurement coordinators, are also responsible for collecting donor data, transmitting that data to UNOS and the transplant centers that will receive the organs, and dealing with families of the deceased donor.[3]

In Germany, offices that mediate activities are called *Organizationzentrale* and are based in transplant centers. Many, but not all, of these offices are associated with the Deutsche Stiftung für Organspende (DSO), a not-for-profit organization that attempts to coordinate national transplant activities. Germany also participates in Eurotransplant (ET), a network organization similar to UNOS. The physician attending a potential donor usually notifies a transplant center directly; possibly he may call ET. The transplant center he notifies may be responsible for a loosely defined capture region; or as is often the case, it may have a longstanding personal or organizational relationship with the physician or the hospital.[4]

Clinical data are transmitted to Eurotransplant to initiate a search for a match. The personnel involved vary, but usually the centers employ physicians as transplant coordinators, called *Transplantation Koordinatoren*. These coordinators work with both donors and recipients but in general do very little hands-on management of the clinical course of the donor. Instead, this is done by the hospital staff. Coordinators usually do not appear on the scene until well after brain death has been confirmed, and, in most cases, after the family has given permission for donation and left the hospital.

In both Germany and the United States, many potential donors come from high-tech urban trauma centers. But many also come from small rural hospitals without the equipment or specialists necessary to diagnose brain death or manage the complicated clinical process. Coordinators trained in dealing with the unique clinical situation of brain-dead bodies have to get to the donor quickly, before organ systems begin to fail or when the opportunity for gaining organs becomes a "problem." After all, brain-dead bodies take up space needed for living patients and are an expensive drain on labor and resources. In the United States, it is common to move brain-dead patients to larger, better-equipped centers, which can perform the extensive tests and provide the clinical management mandated by protocol. German organ procurement centers, however, rarely undergo this sort of expense and difficulty after brain death has been declared, although the diagnosis itself may require either moving the patient or bringing in a neurologist qualified to diagnose brain death.

Wherever the donor is, arrangements must be made to transport the organs, often across great distances. The recipient patient is usually at a transplant center in another part of the country (or, in Europe, possibly in another country). Some are still well enough to live at home and must get to their transplant centers by the time organs become available.

Patients needing a transplant are normally registered at the transplant center where they hope to have the procedure performed. (They are supposed to be registered at only one center.) After screening and acceptance, their names are added to a waiting list.[5] In the United States, UNOS keeps a registry of waiting recipients and takes information about donors as they become available in order to find matches between the two. ET performs this function for several countries in Europe. Information is recorded about the severity of a recipient's illness, the urgency of need (that is, an estimate of how close the recipient is to death), his blood and tissue type, his age and size, the length of time his name has been on the list, complications, and so on. Basic information about the donor (blood type, size, cause of death, key laboratory data) is forwarded to UNOS or ET and compared to profiles from the pool of transplant candidates. Possible matching recipients are selected, based on a mixture of factors: tissue type, size (a small child cannot receive a lung from a 250–pound man), blood type, and other characteristics.

Here, however, the system becomes more complex. Both the system structure and the rules of matching vary by organ. Some organs are center-driven, meaning that transplant centers take turns for their waiting recipients according to a complicated point system. Other organs are patient-driven—that is, the list is based on the situation of individual patients regardless of their transplant center. These systems differ by country; and even within the same country and system, there are wide variations in practice and interpretation of rules.

Once a subset of possible matches has been made, coordinators at the OPO or the Organizationzentrale forward further clinical data about the donor to transplant centers where potential recipients are registered. Based on the clinical picture of the donor as described by the coordinator, transplant surgeons decide if they will accept or reject the offer for their patient. They also weigh other factors that might cause problems, such as risk of infection or disease from the donor and the current status of the intended recipient. Just as important are logistical factors, such as whether a surgical team can be summoned quickly (often in the middle of the night) or if the recipient can get to the clinic. If permission has been given to remove several organs, then multiple transplant center teams become involved.[6]

The coordinator makes all arrangements for the surgical procedure itself. A surgical team from the recipient's transplant center usually retrieves thoracic and abdominal organs. Kidneys are sometimes retrieved by a team close to the donor hospital and then shipped to their destination via ambulance or air transport.[7] Surgeons can still reject an organ at this point if it appears to be damaged or anatomically insufficient in some way. Any tissues to be removed are taken out after the organs, in either the operating room or the morgue. Finally, the body cavity is sewn up, and the body is taken to the morgue and prepared for the funeral home or crematorium.

The chapters in part 2 expand on this brief description. Chapter 6 takes a broad view of infrastructural and organizational elements, including the political and historical influences that have contributed to existing arrangements. Chapter 7 examines how primary workers in organ procurement carry out their work, mediating between global and local activities and concerns. Chapters 8 and 9 focus on the actual procurement procedure, analyzing practices within their many contexts.

Six

Organizing the Procurement and Use of Human Materials

Who controls the organs controls transplant medicine.
(Eurotransplant representative, f.n., June 1994)

The particular form that institutions, organizations, and other social arrangements take cannot be separated from the historical events and cultural notions embedded in everyday postwar, postunification German life. The arrangements for organ procurement and transplantation are relatively public, formal, and institutionalized. Although tissue and cells are often (but not always) procured from the same sources as organs, they have different organizational requirements based on technical needs and constraints as well as legal status and conceptions of the material's nature. Tissue is collected and distributed in a more ad hoc way than organs are, although new technical, economic, and legal developments are encouraging the growth of transnational networks. Materials for research have a legal and moral status different from the status of transplant organs and are collected for specific projects in an informal way that is far less visible to the public.

Organization and work arrangements depend partly on the tasks necessary to do the work, although constraints and unanticipated opportunities may modify these tasks or the ways in which they are carried out. Some modifications involve social and cultural processes at both local and global levels; for example, local changes in policies, events, or social processes can affect and be affected by more global political-economic changes. Such interactions shape the form that these arrangements take.

For many people, perceptions of German institutions are tainted by the memory of the two world wars. Therefore, to have merit, organizations, laws, and practices must not appear to repeat the past. They must seem credible to economic and scientific exchange partners around the world as well as to German citizens at home. In short, medical practices, institutions, and regulations are being reconstructed in much the same way as other facets of German society. Structures, classifications, methods, and procedures are being redesigned to demonstrate that Germany has science and social life under control. "Work," then, not only involves selecting tools, people, and techniques to make the technology function but deals with balancing concerns about moral behavior and the protection of individuals' rights with notions of scientific progress. Meeting the expectations and demands of the global economy must be articulated with the task of reformulating German society.

At the international level, the social domain of human materials technology may seem like a microcosm of EU politics and economic policy. Here also, policymakers are attempting to harmonize structures and policies regarding the use and exchange of human tissue across national borders. Beneath these proposed transnational and national structures lies the assumption that transplantation is a rational science with generalizable practices that can be standardized. When we examine practices at the local level, however, we see how these "universals" are resisted, reinterpreted, or accommodated.

Facilitating Transnational Trade: Organization across Europe

Before a systematic infrastructure was in place, physicians themselves arranged to get cadaveric organs to waiting patients. There was no formal exchange system; organs went to the closest and the sickest.[1] Because preservation techniques were poor, organs had to be implanted as quickly as possible after removal to minimize the amount of natural deterioration.

Still, outcomes were poor; some recipients' bodies rejected donor tissue. Immunological research indicated that human leukocyte antigens (HLA) are key to determining tissue compatibility.[2] This set of antigens exists on the surface of cells in varying combinations. According to proponents of HLA matching theory, the pattern of these six key antigens in the donor should be matched as closely as possible to the recipient's pattern to minimize the risk of tissue reaction. The theory suggests that a best-match system has better outcomes than a system that gives organs to the sickest patients or the ones waiting the longest (Opelz 1992).

In most countries today, matching donor and recipient tissue according to antigen patterns undergirds the system for allocating organs.[3] The supply of human tissue is not ample, and requiring tissue types to be closely matched means that finding the right tissue tool has become more difficult. Thus, it makes sense for large numbers of clinics to cooperate by pooling and exchanging what is available.

To make this system work, a centralized source must capture data, interpret findings, and compare donor data to recipient data. Standardized methods for typing tissue and systematically applying guidelines for sharing are also necessary to ensure that transplant centers play by the same rules. At the same time, centers must be able to communicate data and transport materials quickly over great distances. Some tissues must be processed and stored so that they can be used interchangeably long after the initial collection.

Thus, technologies that use human materials depend on elaborate medical and nonmedical infrastructures. Medical infrastructure includes chemical, mechanical, and electronic technologies for diagnosis, preservation, and processing. Nonmedical infrastructure includes information systems, transport and communications systems, and energy.[4] Ingo Braun and Bernward Joerges (1993) call these nonmedical institutions "second-order technical systems"—that is, systems developed within and superimposed on the frame of existing technical structures and a specific social domain.[5]

Intertransplant, a now-defunct organ-exchange organization that served eastern bloc nations, exemplified the critical nature of this infrastructure.[6] While Intertransplant was effective enough to exchange scholarly and scientific information, it never functioned well for material exchanges because key infrastructural ingredients were missing. Air and ground transport systems were poor, telephone systems did not always work well, and the bureaucracy of crossing borders was overwhelming. Organs were sometimes shipped to Eurotransplant when infrastructural problems prevented their use in Intertransplant countries. Physicians claim, however, to have rarely received organs from ET because of blockades and other political difficulties. According to one East German physician, "the politicians played their games, and the organs were held hostage" (f.n., September 1994). Data I collected from Intertransplant archives supported this claim, although the situation changed quickly after unification: forty-six organs delivered to East German clinics were handled through ET in 1990 compared with fourteen organs the year before unification.

The Intertransplant example shows that large-scale systems require mechanisms to overcome logistical, technological, legal, and social barriers. To begin with, agreed-upon definitions and classifications are essential to facilitating exchange of information and tissue across national, organizational, and cultural boundaries. There must be a common understanding of what the data mean, which data are important, and how tissue must be handled for best results.

Organ Procurement in Europe

The exchange of human materials requires some entity or mechanism that links professional groups and advisory bodies at the international, national, and local levels. In Europe, transnational differences plus the shortage of a desired commodity created an opportunity for developing a supranational registry and exchange organization.

Eurotransplant was founded in 1969 as a not-for-profit organization to perform this role. ET registers both transplant recipients and donors, collects and conveys data, and acts as a professional consortium for education and political advocacy. Contrary to popular perception, ET is not a pan-European organization, nor does it have the authority to mandate local practices within its participating countries: Germany, Austria, Belgium, and the Netherlands.[7] ET members are individual transplant centers that voluntarily participate and provide information. For these clinics, the advantage of belonging to a multinational system is better access to larger pools of donated organs. A greater number and variety of tissue types are more likely to yield an organ that matches a recipient's tissue type and therefore has a better probability of successful grafting. Membership is particularly advantageous for clinics in countries with low rates of donation. Transplant centers in these countries may be more likely to acquire organs from another country through a transnational exchange service than to find an appropriate organ at home.

An image of control and scientific rationality is key to ET's viability as a central coordinating unit. The ET computer system, Pioneer, takes in scientific data about donors and potential recipients (presumably unfiltered by human interpretation), objectively makes its calculations, and produces the best match between organ and needy patient regardless of where in Europe each is located—or so the myth goes. This image of an all-powerful, wise, objective, and benevolent nonhuman agent appears in all transplant publications as well as in all media stories, even the most negative ones. ET itself is often described as an Oz-like center for this computer oracle.

As the physical embodiment of the wizard, the organization conveys symbolic messages that tacitly link information, medical science, transnational politics, and the mythical image of healing and sharing across nations. ET headquarters are located in Leiden, a university town in the Netherlands with a centuries-old reputation as a center for medical science and research. Arriving for a visit, I stepped off the train from Amsterdam and found myself in a rail station directly connected to an enormous hospital complex where ET offices are housed. The walkway leading from this complex was blue and yellow—European Union colors as well as Dutch national colors. The offices themselves are small and resemble the mundane administrative offices of any other enterprise. Yet as ET officers told me, it is important for them to be housed in a medical setting to project a medical image rather than an administrative or business one.

Patients are registered on waiting lists at transplant centers for each type of organ, and clinical data about their condition and tissue type are sent to ET. Information about potential donors is also sent to ET and includes basic data about age, sex, cause of death, and clinical test results. Using rules established by medical committees, workers enter data into the Pioneer system. Organs from potential donors are then allocated according to matching tissue and blood type, body size, and length of time on the waiting list, among other variables. There is considerable negotiation of data, however, which determines how this information is handled.

The use of predetermined rules and procedural guidelines is a way of creating a common "language" through which members can communicate.

Protocols and standards theoretically ease the exchange of materials by eliminating local or specific techniques that might not be acceptable in other places. Still, characteristics of local contexts resist standardization. For example, I often observed German physicians removing organs according to an arduous, craftlike method not used elsewhere.[8] In one case, a Dutch coordinator told me, "You will never see this anymore after a couple of years. Only the Germans do this" (f.n., May 1994).

Translating data and performing procedures across languages create another logistical problem in transnational exchange. For example, a number of Dutch speak German and other languages, but fewer Germans, particularly those from the former GDR, can speak foreign languages, including English (the official language of organ exchange in Europe). This creates difficulties not only in negotiating the exchange of information and arranging the transfer of materials but during procurement procedures themselves. In some of my observations, physicians occasionally resorted to a form of sign language to indicate surgical instruments or request something during a procedure. More than once I was pressed into duty as a translator.

For Germany, belonging to a supranational organization is key to projecting an image of a system under control—crucial in this time of public uncertainty. Organizations involved in organ procurement claim to be entirely transparent to the public.[9] Their structures and rules are portrayed as purely objective, based on scientific facts and medical criteria established by knowledgeable experts both inside and outside of Germany.

With a number of large and active transplant centers, Germany is a powerful member of ET. Several of my respondents stated that Germany formed about two-thirds or more of ET membership. Since the organization's founding, Germany has been strongly represented on the board and on all technical committees. This German bloc was weakened in 1994, when a change in board and committee structures shifted representation and effectively removed the old guard from positions of power. Representation is now organized by organ, and delegates from centers with higher numbers of transplants have more votes (Eurotransplant Foundation 1994: 4).

Because of comparatively low internal donation rates, Germany acquires many organs from outside the country (primarily but not entirely from other ET member countries), while exporting very few. This, of course, creates imbalances in organ circulation, which other participating countries resent.[10] I attended ET meetings in 1992, 1993, and 1994, and the number of anti-German comments seemed to increase each year. Surgeons from other countries were concerned that Germans were taking all the organs. In the words of one surgeon, "Germany is a disaster! They don't donate any organs, and it's just like a sinkhole for the rest of us" (f.n., September 1993).

Some surgeons were disturbed by the power structures in the organization, believing that Germany needed to be kept under control. According to one Dutch surgeon, "we have to break the German cartel" (f.n., September 1993). Another Dutch surgeon told me, "The Germans have to be controlled. Otherwise no one else gets what they need" (f.n., September 1994). And an Austrian surgeon declared, "It's about time we changed the organization [of ET]. Those Germans have been running things too long, and now we want to have our say" (f.n., September 1994). Their resentment and mistrust parallel European sentiments about Germans more generally as concern grows about the nation's growing economic, military, and geographic presence and concomitant power.

There was considerable speculation among ET member representatives that Germany would drop out of ET, especially since one version of the country's proposed transplant law instituted a central organization to coordinate data and activities. If a presumed consent law were passed, they reasoned, the number of donors within Germany would increase. The country would thus become more self-sufficient, no longer obliged to abide by ET rules. The fact is, however, that Germany needs the legitimacy and symbolic power of belonging to a transnational scientific effort. The idea of creating a centralized authority and then claiming rights to the disposal of citizens' bodies has a far too familiar ring.

Tissue Procurement in Europe

A wide variety of tissues are used for replacement or reconstruction—primarily bones, corneas, and heart valves. Most tissues may be procured up to twenty-four hours after death (or more, according to some sources) because they are less vascularized than organs (or not vascularized at all): that is, they have no direct blood supply and therefore are not oxygen dependent. Thus, they do not need to come from brain-dead patients. Tissue procurement activities involve a number of separate organizations and personnel with varying skill, education, and status levels.

Organization of European tissue procurement activities is uneven, historically surrounding interests in specific tissues. Examples are the Dutch Burn Foundation (supporting skin donation) and the European Skeletal-Muscular Foundation (which supports the donation of bone, bone components, tendons, and other structural tissues). Procurement has been largely performed within clinics for specific and immediate use; stockpiling inventory for future use or for large demand, as in the event of a major disaster, is not routinely practiced. In recent years, however, demand has increased beyond what individual organizations and clinics are able to supply.

One option was to take the Eurotransplant model for organs and apply it to tissues: centralizing, standardizing, and controlling procurement and distribution would not only meet increased demand but expand ET's base at a time of shrinking organ—and thus income—supply. A centralized organization could administer the increased regulations and data necessary for transplantable tissues as well as promote and pay for procurement, serve as an efficient exchange system, and enlarge the pool of available materials. Profit could come from registry fees, and operations support from private and public funds. Banks could also turn over inventory more quickly and lower costs.

To this end, BioImplant Services (BIS) was created in 1988 as ET's spinoff not-for-profit tissue procurement organization. The link is made explicit in the BIS information brochure (BioImplant Services 1994b). Its theme is building bridges, and in bold type on the first page is this statement: "Bridging between fields of organ and tissue transplantation is vital." In the Netherlands, that idea is being put into action through combined tissue and organ procurement protocols. Local practices in Germany, however, are intended to keep the two domains quite separate.

BIS functions as a tissue donor registry and exchange organization. By contracting with tissue banks for administrative services, it works to expand its network of tissue providers (hospitals and clinics) and improve the efficiency of placement in contracted banks. BIS develops quality and safety standards and supports scientific studies regarding processing, analysis, and use of materials.

Quality and safety standards (modeled after U.S. good manufacturing practices and Food and Drug Administration recommendations) are intended for use throughout Europe as a way of standardizing and controlling procedures and products as legislation changes. The purpose is clear:

Building bridges between European tissue banks and transplant surgeons is a prime goal for BIS. As the demand for tissue transplantation throughout Europe continues to grow, it will be essential for tissue banks to cooperate across national borders. This cooperation will depend upon the confidence between banks that similar tissue quality and safety standards are being observed. (BioImplant Services 1994b: 20)

Around the world, regulation of tissue procurement and distribution is increasing, particularly because of threats of HIV infection and concerns about unregulated commercial markets. Scandals in Germany (discussed in chapter 5) have added to pressures for regulation. But various European countries define and classify tissues differently. While most call them "biologicals," in Germany tissues fall into the category of *Arzneimittel* (pharmaceuticals), mostly comprised of man-made products. Such classification differences create interesting challenges for standardization. Eurovalid, a consulting firm specializing in standardizing manufacturing and clinical practices, validation, and quality assurance, has already implemented good manufacturing practices (GMPs) in two tissue banks. Standard operating procedures have been adopted at the same institutions to specify materials and reagents used and govern processing procedures. These measures, borrowed directly from manufacturing industries, are meant to create reproducible practices that can be applied across the wide variety of skill levels, technical capabilities, national regulations, and professional groups involved in procuring and exchanging tissues in Europe—a tall order.

With so many legal, political, ethical, technical, and national borders involved, there are tremendous difficulties in gaining compliance with such standards. These logistical problems are made more difficult by the ambiguity involved in attempting to combine items that are simultaneously human and object. I asked several people if standardizing procedures would also create problems of liability and warranty. One tissue bank representative told me:

Well, we want to be liable. We want to be responsible for what we're doing. But we cannot give a warranty, no. That's in the Creator's hands. He has created this tissue. We have only checked it. Like the cornea: does it have regular cells? Does it have at least 72,300 cells per millimeter? We want to be responsible for the processing work, yes. (f.n., June 1994)

The representative affirms the sacred nature of human remains. Rather than simply constraining what people can do with the material, however, its sacred nature presents a unique opportunity. If God has made the material and it is thus both natural and sacred, then the distributor cannot be blamed or held liable for flaws, inefficacy, or problems.

In Germany, tissue procurement efforts are sparse, and few tissue banks exist. Instead, material is ordered from European or American sources or collected by clinics for specific in-house use. As with organs, Germany shows a disparity between the number of tissues procured and the number transplanted. For example, compared with other BIS members, in 1993 it provided 5 percent of the pool of actual cornea donors but performed 32.6 percent of all corneal transplants. In 1994 it provided 14.2 percent of cornea donors but performed 49.6 percent of transplants. By comparison, in 1994 the Netherlands procured 80 percent of donor corneas but transplanted only 47 percent (BioImplant Services 1994a: 27). Similarly, in 1994, 43.1 percent of all heart valve allografts shipped from BIS contract banks went to German clinics.[11]

Future Trends

As various EU organizations become more actively involved, transnational organ and tissue exchange will become even more challenging. The Council of Europe is already examining standards for procurement, tissue typing, and exchange, assigning committees to develop standards of practice to be sent to the European parliament. In 1995 the council sponsored an intensive course for coordinators to enhance professional skills and promote standardized techniques. The involvement of new actors will increase the problems of economic and political coordination, further dilute old power bases in medicine, and demand new organizational forms to deal with additional layers of regulation and bureaucracy.

In addition, more nonmember countries want to share the pool of available materials. ET's 1992 annual report documents this change, calling for deliberations to consider how to handle allocation to nonmember clinics both within and outside the EU. A growing number of patients want to be on transplant waiting lists in Europe as well as in their home countries, believing they will thus have a better chance for receiving an organ. This is leading to a type of health tourism common in other medical services where facilities, equipment, or specialists are concentrated in wealthy countries or those with fewer restrictions on certain procedures.

I visited several German transplant centers that have already set up their own consortium agreements with specific eastern European clinics, primarily in the Czech Republic and Poland. In exchange for working with physicians from these countries to establish new transplant centers and train surgeons, German surgeons receive organs from the clinics. These agreements—and organs—are separate from ET arrangements and are not reported in ET statistics. They are a creative if problematic solution to the severe shortage problem in Germany. Transplant physicians told me that materials are easier to acquire in the east. They believe that, compared to Germans, people are more compliant and less resistant to donating organs and tissues and that physicians are happy to exchange organs for skills and technology. At the same time, German transplant centers are not compelled to make such arrangements transparent to the public.

Facilitating Procurement at Home: Organization in Germany
According to the many German coordinators and surgeons I interviewed, each transplant center has locally established policies and procedures allowing them the ability to participate in ET exchange while maintaining flexibility as independent operators. I now consider the multiple levels of organization and disjuncture within Germany itself.

Organ Procurement in Germany
There are more than forty transplant centers in Germany specializing in different organs. The number fluctuates as new centers open (mostly in the east) and smaller ones are forced out of operation by competition with large centers.[12] Most, but not all, transplant centers participate as members in the Deutsche Stiftung für Organspende (DSO), the German foundation for organ donation, a not-for-profit organization handling procurement and maintaining donor and recipient data in cooperation with ET. The DSO pays procurement coordinator salaries at member centers and covers equipment, materials, transportation, and other administrative costs associated with procuring organs for transplantation. Instead of working through the DSO, German transplant centers can opt to deal with ET independently, and some have also attempted alternative regional or local arrangements.

The DSO was formed in 1984 by the Kuratorium für Hemodialyse (KfH), a professional physician-based association that has expanded its interests from dialysis to kidney transplantation, "recogniz[ing] the increasing costs to society of maintaining patients on dialysis" (f.n., September 1992; Kuratorium für Hemodialyse 1993: 18). This growing concern has coincided with a decline in profitability in dialysis, increased competition from other dialysis firms, and the advent of health care financing reform, all of which contributed to the expansion to transplant activities.

Although the DSO and KfH have separate legal structures, they are governed by the same board, and the DSO's funding comes primarily from KfH. Also involved is the Arbeitskreis Organspende (Committee for Organ Donation), which KfH founded in 1979 and funds to promote organ donation. Among the members of the Arbeitskreis are the national German medical association, public and private insurance funds, patient advocacy organizations, and the federal minister for health. A professional organization, the Arbeitsgemeinschaft der Deutschen Transplantation Zentren e.V. (Society for German Transplant Centers), is concerned with medical and scientific affairs and issues guidelines for practice.[13]

The DSO is supposed to promote donation to the public and (as I learned at a member meeting) is violently opposed to allowing coordinators or centers to pursue such activities on their own. In reality, however, the organization does virtually no public promotion other than provide pamphlets in dialysis clinics and at occasional health fairs. It collects media stories and disseminates them each month to transplant coordinators but offers no analysis or rebuttal to negative media stories. Despite criticism from transplant surgeons who believe that the organization should focus on public education rather than what they see as interference in medical affairs, the DSO continues to concentrate on operations and professional concerns.

According to coordinators and transplant surgeons, the DSO has no real authority over medical or administrative practice (for example, where or how organs are selected or used). Furthermore, even though the DSO pays salaries and expenses for member transplant offices, coordinators are normally responsible to another department (usually urology or the heart or liver service) within local transplant centers.

The DSO pays participating donor hospitals about two thousand marks per organ procured, although this figure is negotiable. One coordinator told me his center received 2,500 marks for kidneys alone and 3,500 marks if more than one organ was procured from a donor (f.n., July 1994). Another said his center received five thousand marks each for livers and hearts (f.n., June 1994).[14] Still, these sums are very low in light of the costs, labor, and trouble involved—hardly enough to induce hospitals to procure for income, contrary to popular horror stories and urban myths.

The DSO operates an extensive computer information network (known as TIS) through which associate transplant centers register recipients and donors. Key data on patients are then passed on to Eurotransplant. Although the computer system functions as a gatekeeper, data are extremely difficult to extract for analyses, and the program is complicated to operate. There is no mechanism for collecting statistics or analyzing data (for example, to find out why organs were not donated or not used), nor is information tracked (other than basics such as blood type, weight, and tissue type results) to characterize donors. Many functions duplicate ET's Pioneer system, but the two systems did not link well at the time of my research.

Because kidneys were the first organs to be transplanted with any frequency, the DSO was once governed mainly by kidney specialists. Since then, the organization has grown rapidly in size and bureaucracy. Now that surgeons are transplanting a wider variety of organs (primarily hearts and livers in Germany), new professional medical groups have become involved. With more complicated payment and allocation systems, powerful nonmedical players, such as insurance funds and patient rights groups, have also joined the game. Thus, the roles of individual clinics, the DSO, and other interest groups have shifted.

Today, the DSO expends much effort on garnering power and centralizing authority. It receives a large amount of federal funding for research on new technologies and scientific studies. Its primary project is a large longitudinal study intended to demonstrate definitively that tissue matching for HLA antigens is essential to good transplant outcomes for all organs. Adopting this system as a basis of exchange not only for kidneys but for other organs would require the establishment of a central organizing body to manage tissue matching. DSO board members and lawyers have lobbied for writing "a central organizing body" into transplant legislation. Gaining formal authority would solidify the DSO's ability to centralize because it would be the only organization in a position to disseminate information and to implement and control technologies.

Meanwhile, many coordinators, hospital physicians, and insurers resent the immense cost of operating the DSO, especially since they see no visible results in terms of increased donations or greater efficiency.[15] Moreover, as health reform initiatives squeeze profits in the dialysis industry, KfH has less money available for DSO operations; the organization was 50 million marks in the red in 1994 (DSO staff member, personal communication, 1994). Costs are spread among participating dialysis centers in the KfH and transplant centers, which are being asked to underwrite more operating expenses. Dialysis physicians wonder why they should bear the costs of transplantation activities, and clinics questioning the high charges for organ procurement services want to see a direct cost reckoning. Transplant centers pay the DSO twelve thousand marks per transplant for organs and services (about $8,160 at the time of my research).

Despite the DSO's increased presence in negotiating financial and organizational schemes, practitioners (surgeons, in particular) deny that the organization plays a major role in practice. They see its role as coordinating procurement logistics rather than influencing medical practice or technical affairs. Consider the following conversations:

> *LH:* Could you tell me something about the German system [of procurement]?
>
> *Liver surgeon:* (laughs) System? There is no German system. There are only *systems* that are in Germany. (f.n., August 1992)

Another respondent even discounted the DSO's administrative and financial roles:

> *LH:* How would you describe the German system of procurement?
>
> *Coordinator:* What do you mean, system of procurement? We are all members of Eurotransplant, of course. Is that what you mean? But we here have our way of doing things, and then Berlin has theirs, Kiel theirs, and then of course there's Bavaria, which is another story entirely. We all know what each other does—how we do things. And we understand each other. But there's no national system, if that's what you mean.

LH: What about the DSO? I thought they were the national. . . .

Another coordinator: (interrupts) They have no role. They can't tell us what to do. Sure, they pay the salaries and buy equipment, but we don't let them interfere with the way we do things here. (f.n., January 1994)

To reinforce this perception of local and regional independence and control, some people argued that professional medical knowledge took precedence over administrative or nonmedical knowledge:

LH: So you're saying that Germany has a nationally organized agency that pays the salaries of procurement professionals, pays hospitals for organs and receives income from insurance funds, provides equipment for procurements and transport for materials, plus there is a national computerized system through which all donors and recipients must be registered and categorized, plus there are two professional organizations that oversee technical, legal, and ethical problems—yet you say there is no systematic organization for procuring materials throughout Germany?

Kidney surgeon: Well, *we* are systematic, and I'm sure other centers are, too. But these organizations we're talking about—they can only make suggestions. This DSO, for example, is in Frankfurt, not here. And besides, it's run by nonphysicians. They have nothing to say about medical matters. (f.n., February 1994)

These early encounters with procurement professionals puzzled me. Not only were people reluctant to describe any organization, institution, practices, or individuals outside their own institution and nearby geographic regions, but they also consistently belittled the validity of all supraorganizational entities, including the federal legislature.[16] But when I considered these responses in the context of German history, they said a great deal about the importance of geography, identity, and medical autonomy in German society. Practices and institutions are, after all, inseparable from local history and culture. In Germany, we must consider not the history of a nation or a "national style" so much as the history of politically bound regions, local and regional identities, and the reconstruction of the medical organization in light of its past. It is this background that must be understood in order to organize and control the exchange of human material.

Geography and History: Trade Routes, Political Divisions, and the Exchange of Body Parts

At the time of my research, the DSO was just beginning to plan regionalization of services in ways similar to U.S. organization of procurement. Regionalization makes operations more efficient because some equipment and services can be shared. In the United States, assigned coordinators can cover targeted geographic areas, developing stronger ties and trust relationships with individual hospitals, with the goal of increasing the number of donors reported. The United States is formally organized along these lines, sharing personnel, expenses, and administration within exactly defined borders.

While clinics generally follow the protocol guidelines of professional medical associations and ET guidelines for exchanging organs, I quickly learned that each clinic in Germany has its own methods and system. I observed that in several parts of Germany clinics have made separate agreements with each other to coordinate efforts in the procurement and exchange of materials. Made among clinic physicians and administrators, these agreements exist entirely outside of ET and the DSO.

Forming regional cooperatives decreases the intense competition between clinics that are vying for the same donors. It also connotes an informal and tacit agreement to keep organs in the region first before sharing with the larger German or ET pool. As one can imagine, these are not formal or public efforts. Coordinators were extremely hesitant to talk about these arrangements, although a few quietly slipped me maps or planning guides with clinic locations listed.

Where are these territories of exchange? In contrast to what one might expect, they do not fall along state or east-west lines. They are not related to the movement of certain physicians to new clinics and are not consistently related to personal connections among physicians. They cut across state borders, some of which have different regulations that might affect medical practice. Instead, plotting the cooperative arrangements reveals patterns remarkably similar to ancient political and trade routes.[17] One region includes Bremen and Hamburg in the west and Rostock to the east, encompassing the northern areas of Lower Saxony and Mecklenburg.[18] This was a stable and profitable Hanseatic trade route that functioned between the twelfth and the sixteenth centuries. In 1996, clinics in Dresden, Halle, and Leipzig in the central eastern part of Germany formalized a relationship, another area historically linked through trade and cultural exchange (Matschke et al. 1997).

Kiel, in the northwest corner, stayed out of this arrangement but continues to cooperate with Scandiatransplant, the transplant organization for Scandinavia. The northwest region of Germany has at various times in history been part of Denmark, lying outside the Holy Roman Empire that encompassed most of what is now Germany. The former Prussian stronghold of territories around Berlin and Brandenburg forms another region. Yet another is in the southwest corner, covering Heidelberg, Stuttgart, part of the Rhineland, and Baden-Württemberg up to Frankfurt but excluding the far southern town of Freiburg, just an hour south of Heidelberg. The Swabian League formed a trade bridge in the southwest between Tyrol and Burgundy and became a mainstay of political order through the 1500s, and the Rhenish League in this area held a strong monopoly on cloth and metalwork. Bavaria, for many years a separate state, not surprisingly forms its own region and has a rather formalized system by comparison. The striking obduracy of such regional ties and identity is one of many reasons why new political boundaries such as the European Union may be only partially successful in their attempts to create supraordinate governance and standardized ways of seeing the world.

I turn now to another artificial boundary, the line between East and West Germany, which created deep divisions within a relatively short period that have had dramatic effects on practices and policies, both in medicine and in other aspects of society. The ways in which identity has evolved have directly affected medical work: how it is organized, the philosophy of sharing resources such as human materials, and the ways in which uses of the body are conceptualized.

The organization and administration of organ procurement was handled quite differently in East and West Germany. East German transplantation was centralized in Berlin, with some procedures at Rostock, Halle, and Jena. Transplant services were extremely centralized: one of the few (but richly

supported) high-tech medical services.[19] Although socialist medicine focused on prevention and the polyclinic system, transplant medicine offered
an opportunity to participate internationally and opened doors to related areas of research, such as immunology. Another reason for the preeminence
of transplant medicine was Professor Maurice Mebel, an East German kidney surgeon trained in the Soviet Union, who was one of the first to perform transplants in the GDR. He was also a member of the Zentralkommittee
of the Communist party, which decided political and social affairs. He held
extraordinary power because of his dual position as respected medical professional with close ties to the Soviet Union and as political leader with the
interests of medicine at heart.

At reunification, the two systems had to be joined. The Widerspruch-
lösung and Leichenoffnung laws were immediately terminated because
westerners considered it improper and even immoral not to inform families about the use of bodies after death. (This reaction seems ironic today,
given the presumed consent law proposed in the 1990s.) Many university-
based physicians lost their jobs during the overview process that exposed
individuals with Stasi connections. Still, some of these physicians remain,
and ties and loyalties between them and outlying clinics have not changed.

The DSO overhauled procedures, record keeping, organization, and personnel in the former GDR's university clinics. It purchased equipment and
supplies and set up offices in key eastern locations, although salaries for
coordinators in the east are only 80 percent of those in the west. There were
even more basic infrastructure problems to contend with. For example, one
heart patient was required to live in the clinic for more than two months
after his transplant because he had no phone at home and could not be monitored by the usual clinic telecommunications (f.n., September 1992).[20]

Because of rapid changes, new organization, and the removal of a law
that clearly stated what was allowable and how to proceed, medical personnel worked in a gray zone for the first few years after reunification. Physicians were not sure what to do. Today, lack of philosophical agreement,
mutual blame for problems, and cultural stereotypes continue to plague both
sides and hinder cooperation. While I often heard westerners complain
about the east's poor quality of organs and practices, I saw in records from
individual clinics that, proportionately, more organs are procured from eastern clinics than from the much larger number of clinics in the west. This

has created some friction: most procured organs are given to West German clinics or European clinics; the east's patients do not receive an equivalent number of organs in return. The situation has created an image of the east as little more than a supplier to wealthier centers in the west, getting short shrift in return—an image that parallels other forms of industrial production.

Tissue Procurement in Germany

Although there have been increasing efforts to centralize and co-ordinate tissue procurement and distribution transnationally, activities remain fragmented. This is especially true in Germany, where there are few banks for processing and storage. Those that do exist function primarily to serve the clinic where materials have been collected; they are not store-houses for exchange.

Since human implants are classified as pharmaceuticals in Germany, they are supposed to be regulated in the same way as drugs. This means that anyone procuring and distributing materials must have a *Herstellung* (a business permit and registration) and agree to follow drug quality control and other regulatory procedures. The authorities, however, have always looked the other way, allowing tissues and organs to be implanted with the assumption that material is used in the clinic where it was procured. Because there have been no formally organized tissue banks in Germany to procure or receive materials from numerous sources and distribute them to other us-ers, the situation has never been challenged. Respondents told me there was a long-standing and well-organized tacit agreement with the authorities whereby procurement of organs and tissues was largely ignored. As one respondent explained, "who else was there to do it, and how would it get done otherwise?" (f.n., August 1994).

Ironically, a new Berlin bank, the Central Tissue Bank, upset this arrange-ment by following the rules literally and formally applying for a business license. The bank was formed in the wake of a scandal involving a for-profit bank in the same location, and it wanted to do things properly. Instead, it caught the authorities and the Berlin senate off guard, forcing them to make other clinics comply. Suddenly all clinics procuring tissue had to identify themselves, their procedures, and what they procure and apply for a license. This meant they would have to hire regulatory personnel to establish and oversee a quality-control program, just as if the clinic were manufacturing drugs—a very expensive and difficult proposition. Otherwise, banks would be restricted to using material only within their own clinic. As a result, a number of valves and other tissues would have to be thrown away rather than being sent to other clinics. Longstanding informal arrangements between clinics were disrupted. New arrangements are now being formed similar to the agreements for organ exchange with countries in eastern Europe.

Well-publicized scandals about tissue collection have made tissue banks cautious about sharing information or making their activities public. Adding to their somewhat gothic image, tissue banks are well hidden from the public. The Berlin heart valve bank, for example, is located in an industrial part of the former East Berlin, far away from its mother clinic in the west, in a hundred-year-old factory building set well off the main street. A bone bank associated with the Charité Clinic in the former East Berlin is located in the basement of a building tucked in a complex of now unused GDR official buildings away from the main clinic campus. Names are often changed from "bank" to "laboratory," or the name of an associated hospital department is used, as in Charité's bone bank, which operates under the name Institut für Transfusionmedizin und Immunohaematologie (Institute for Transfusion Medicine and Hematology). This masks the activity and lends a scientific connotation. The managers I spoke to felt that the public would view the idea of banking or stockpiling materials with suspicion, if not horror, especially in light of recent scandals. A western employee of one bank that was moved to the east suggested that if the facility were called a tissue bank, people would try to rob it. This comment was typical of several I heard from westerners, stereotyping the stupidity and dangerous behavior of easterners.

Human tissue materials are also collected for research, which is forbidden by German transplantation guidelines unless the patient granted specific permission during her lifetime.[21] There is a tacit assumption that if material is taken, it must be used in the same clinic from which it was taken. Guidelines, however, differ widely by city and region. In response to the continuing practice of selling cadaver materials to commercial organizations, which periodically creates a public storm, the health minister warned hospitals in 1993 that materials should not be sold for profit.

Most coordinators told me that they never asked to take material for research because they expected families to find this request offensive.

Coordinator: Of course, you can use tissue for research, but it's tricky. You can't ask the family for parts for research, and you can't ask, "If we take it and can't use it for transplants, can we use it for research?" because they will be suspicious and think you are selling it or experimenting. So we just tell them if they ask.

   LH: Do they ever ask?

Coordinator: No, never. (f.n., April 1994)

Pathologists also presume that the removal of certain tissues is considered normal procedure: "these are tiny, unimportant pieces of tissue that might be removed anyway during the course of an autopsy" (f.n., April 1994). Coordinators consistently deny that tissues or organs are taken for research without permission; but while observing organ procurements, I witnessed removals for research on several occasions. Surgical nurses told me such removals occur routinely. The nurses object to the practice because they feel it is wrong to take more than what is permitted. One surgical nurse verbally objected when an additional section of ureter was removed for a study, but the coordinator and other surgeons told her she was being foolish and obstructive. The coordinator on the case related the story:

One time a surgeon took several centimeters more of a ureter than he needed for the kidney. They were doing a study on stenosis of ureters in his hospital. The surgical nurse said, "Did you see that? He took more than he was supposed to. He shouldn't be using that." But the family said yes to the kidneys, and the ureter belongs to the kidneys as far as I'm concerned. Nurses get so hysterical and so literal about these things—it really causes problems. (f.n., May 1994)

As we can see, it is relatively simple to collect materials when a body is already open and material is being removed: surgeons often use the situation to justify taking an extra bit of tissue, such as a ureter or an unused portion of spleen. Another research source are organs removed for transplantation that are rejected or otherwise not used, despite supposedly strict regulations about returning unused parts to the body cavity. Several respondents admitted that organs were removed and taken to a transplant center and then never used for transplantation.

Global and Local Organization: A Summary

Technologies that use human tissue depend on an elaborate infrastructure of medical and nonmedical institutions, transport and communications technologies, materials science, and a variety of medical technologies to acquire, process, transport, store, and use these organic materials. They are equally dependent on legal and economic arrangements with authorities at local, national, and international levels to obtain and use available material efficiently. By participating in supranational systems of exchange, Germany is drawn into the global economy of a successful and profitable high-technology industry that could lead to many spinoff industries. There is another benefit: this official, visible link to international standardized science and scientific procedures grants Germany a legitimacy outside the German medical profession, which continues to be plagued by mistrust. Considering Germany's historical and political context, this legitimacy is critical. Because the public is wary of German medicine, especially after the scandals mentioned in chapter 5, images of globally accepted technologies give the use of human bodies greater credence as well.

The United States and some other countries have created a structure with freestanding organizations independent of either transplant centers or donor hospitals, staffed by nonmedical and medical personnel, to create an image of objectivity. In contrast, Germany uses hospital-based physicians to procure materials, directly connecting procurement to the ultimate use of materials. In the opinion of most of the coordinators I interviewed, this approach shows the public that materials are used for medicine and science, not for suspicious purposes. The paradox is that an image of *medical*, not separate nonmedical systems of control, is key to showing that science rather than the state or other interests has jurisdiction over the fate of human bodies.

At the same time, physicians want local control over donated organs. The most obvious reason is to be able to use resources for their own patients, increasing the number of organs transplanted and marks deposited. There are other cultural elements involved as well, including resistance to a centralized, national core of authority and the creation of networks that follow the lines of historical cooperative regions. Multiple layers of identities—local, east-west, European, professional specialty, and others—affect transactions at all levels, including official and unofficial policy.

German transplant medicine is caught in a conundrum: to fully participate in this profitable industry (considered in most other nations to be "miracle of life" technology), the country needs a well-oiled, progressive organization. Yet the image of a formalized, centralized machine created specifically to collect substances from the dead is particularly threatening in Germany, where physicians still struggle to distance medicine from the past. The hesitancy to collect tissue for banking or research shows how organ transplantation physicians work to distance themselves and their activities from past practices regarding human experimentation and to identify with the high-tech and more immediately recognizable medical miracle.

Following organs and tissues through various levels of organization helps us recognize the transnational, national, and local connections that link human materials technologies to other political and social concerns. For these technologies to proceed, infrastructural, technical, and cultural elements must be carefully articulated at global and local levels. Yet the articulations are necessarily contingent, changing under shifting conditions. Thus, standardized methods and structures intended to make exchanges across organizational, national, and cultural borders more efficient and routine depend upon negotiations that make them more singular and customized. In the next chapters, I show how such customizing takes place as I follow organs through specific practices of exchange and processing.

Seven

Local Practice

Coordinators and Surgeons

Interpretations of what human materials are, of what value they are (and to whom) are not simply matters of abstract moral reasoning but of how participants build practices around them. Techniques, medical theories, and moral guidelines are all constructed by individuals who bring values, interests, experiences, and knowledge to the field. In this chapter, I introduce the principal participants who influence practices around human materials most directly—namely, the medical professionals who collect and process the materials. Their work involves both the literal hands-on work of managing the bodies themselves and the organizational work discussed in chapter 6.

Procuring Organs

In Germany, organ procurement activities are located within transplant centers themselves, unlike the United States, where procurement organizations are independent and located outside of hospitals. Since the clinic may or may not be associated with the Deutsches Stiftung für Organspende (DSO), the form of organization, level of authority, and type of personnel differ. In smaller transplant clinics, one person may have to perform all roles; but large clinics may have several staff members with more specialized roles, including a coordinator and perhaps another person (usually medically trained) to do administrative and clerical work.[1]

Unlike coordinators in the United States and some European countries, German coordinators are almost all physicians (and almost all male). A small number are nurses with intensive care experience or other medically trained personnel. Several transplant surgeons told me that it is preferable to have a physician as coordinator because this is medical work and nonphysicians are not as qualified. They also felt that only physicians are qualified to talk to patients' families. Having physicians in this role legitimates this type of work with the dead. The role relates tissue removal to high-tech medicine, distancing it from morgue work or human experimentation work.

The use of physicians as coordinators is also related to the extremely hierarchical nature of German medicine: level of responsibility, status, title, and rank are carefully noted in everyday social relations. Among my respondents, for example, it was common for physicians to call other physicians *Kollegen* (colleagues), distinguishing them from nonphysicians—*Mitarbeitern* (co-workers). One coordinator told me of a physician who wanted information about donor protocols but asked first if the coordinator was a Kollege or a Mitarbeiter. Upon learning that the coordinator was not a physician, he asked to speak with a doctor, even though the coordinator had been in charge of all donor procedures for some years.

Transplant coordinators have relatively low status in German medicine. Often the position is a rotation requirement for a year or two before junior physicians are allowed on staff in a more permanent position. As a result of the current oversupply of physicians in Germany, positions in clinics are extremely competitive. Two respondents admitted that they were promised a position at a hospital if they committed to doing the coordinator's job first. Often coordinators are required to do scut work for another department, such as nephrology, or for a higher-status physician in another department. Many young physicians take this opportunity to do the research required in Germany for advanced qualifications, especially since the low number of donors means that actual donor-related work time is minimal. In some centers the job may be only part time; in others the work may be divided into clerical and clinical positions. Coordinators work in cramped, shared offices, and nonphysicians often get little clerical help or financial support for professional activities, such as attending Eurotransplant or professional meetings.[2]

For coordinators who are not physicians, this work represents a step up from the very low-status position of nursing or other health care professions. Still, many people describe negative effects of the work on personal and collegial relationships due to poor public opinion of organ donation. For this reason, coordinators often identify themselves with the implantation end of transplant work rather than the explantation end. Occasionally, nonphysician coordinators attempt to professionalize the work by creating training programs or a certification process akin to those in other European countries and the United States. But so far all these attempts have failed due to lack of support from physician supervisors. In the eyes of the DSO, these efforts compete with the organization's authority and attempt to centralize activities.

In both Germany and the United States, nonphysician coordinators see the work as increasing their status and autonomy. Unlike coordinators in Germany, American procurement coordinators are primarily female nurses with intensive care experience. In both countries, coordinators who were previously nurses often wanted a change from intensive care, saying the work was too routine and that their new job allows independence and variety. American respondents told me the job was "more professional" or "more like management." German respondents who were not physicians described the job as higher status—"a little more equal relationship to the physicians" (f.n., 1992, 1994).

Coordinators in Organizationzentralen participate in activities with both donors and recipients, although the ultimate responsibility for patients lies with the transplant surgeon. In Germany the degree to which procurement and transplantation are integrated is illustrated by the fact that many donor offices keep photos of potential recipients on file along with their medical records. When I asked why they kept photos, respondents replied that photos give staff an identity and add a human face to names on the waiting list. Occasionally, a photo serves as a "before" picture to be compared to an "after" picture. In the United States, this practice would be considered unethical— with the charge that another type of matching might be going on, based on physical appearance or a more personal connection with particular recipients.

Potential donors are reported to the Organizationzentrale by either an intensive care physician, the *Station Arzt* (physician in charge of the intensive care unit), or a head nurse. In the GDR, clinics were required to report all potential donors. In some areas there were strong ties between physicians at outlying clinics and large university clinics in centers such as Berlin, Jena, and Rostock. Since the recent controversy, however, physicians in both eastern and western Germany are increasingly hesitant to report potential donors. In some cities, opposition groups have posted signs at the homes of neurologists and other physicians associated with transplantation, using slogans strikingly similar to those used in the American anti-abortion movement: "This physician murders patients."

Coordinators also reported an increasing aggressiveness, as they called it, from families of brain-dead patients. Even relatives of other intensive care patients who were not brain dead said to physicians: "We are paying attention—we will supervise you! You will get no organs from us!" (f.n., December 1993).

After being notified, coordinators help to manage the clinical course of the donor until surgical teams arrive to begin the procurement procedure; that is, they must maintain the brain-dead body in a stable state so that minimal damage to tissue will occur. The Station Arzt is ultimately in charge, but even that physician may not be trained specifically to deal with this unique situation. Coordinators also make arrangements for tissue typing the donor, coordinate the surgery, and take care of logistics related to getting the procurement team to the site.

Additionally, the coordinator is responsible for conveying information to transplant centers and negotiating decisions to accept or reject the organs, organizing the teams from transplant centers who will come to procure the organs and tissues (explantation teams), scheduling the operating room, and handling further disposal of the body. Physician coordinators in Germany may assist in the actual surgical removal of organs if, as in many small rural towns, the appropriate operating room staff cannot be summoned during the night, when most of these procedures occur.

Occasionally, coordinators must also interact with the police or notify coroners and negotiate with them about what may be done to the body.[3] They arrange tissue typing with local or distant typing laboratories, work with intensive care staff, and deal with the donor's family. These tasks may also entail phoning pathologists, neurologists, and other physicians in the middle of the night; pressuring the laboratory for prompt results; and acting as diplomat and mediator between the hospital where the donor is located and transplant centers.

Coordinators in both the United States and Germany often have a phone at each ear. They are constantly writing notes and negotiating time and space for teams from various transplant centers and local staff who need the bed in the intensive care unit for other patients. Coordinators are constantly located at the intersection of a variety of participants, each of whom has separate and sometimes conflicting interests. They are usually the first to be blamed if things do not go smoothly.

The following excerpt from my field notes gives a sense of procurement's rapid pace, confusing and complicated communications, and necessary negotiations. I have used a pseudonym for confidentiality (f.n., June 1994).

The procedure is scheduled for 16:30. The liver team has to come from far away, so Michael (the coordinator) calls a nearby large transplant center to see if its team will do the liver explantation as a courtesy. The liver would then be shipped to the appropriate center. The nearby center refuses because it does not have its own recipient for the liver.[4]

14:16 The liver transplant center (L-1) calls, and Michael explains how to get to the clinic where the donor is: by air to the largest nearby city, then by ambulance for another half-hour. Michael is worried about rush-hour traffic and urges the team to come sooner than they had planned. The L-1 staff member on the phone asks if the operation could be put off to give the team more time. He estimates arrival at 17:30.

14:20 Michael calls Eurotransplant to say that one of the major heart centers in Germany (H-1) is probably willing to take the heart. Eurotransplant does not respond to this information. While Michael is on the phone, another line rings: H-1 asking for more information. The intended recipient has an infection, so "das Herz hängt in dem Luft," meaning that everything is uncertain (literally, "the heart hangs in the air"). At this point, the physician in charge of intensive care enters the room, asking Michael exactly how many people will be coming and how soon they will get here. He pressures Michael to get the donor into the operating room quickly (and out of the intensive care unit).

14:40 Michael orders transport for the kidney retrieval team.

14:48 Eurotransplant calls. It has offered the heart to a second heart center in another country (H-2), but the center's team cannot be at the clinic until 18:30. (Apparently H-1 has declined the offer without notifying Michael directly.) Michael asks Eurotransplant to offer the heart to a third transplant center because he does not want to delay the start time. He is worried about upsetting the local staff and needs to coordinate heart removal with removal of other organs.

14:55 The unit physician comes into the room again, asking again about timing. Michael assures him that the procedures will start on time. The physician is pleased that L-1 is coming, saying, "They will not cause problems for us."

15:05 A third heart center (H-3) calls to get more information about the donor to decide if it will accept the heart. (Apparently, Eurotransplant has offered the heart to both H-2 and H-3.)

15:20 L-1 calls. The team's arrival time will be 17:00.

15:30 Michael is still arranging transport and making calls to transplant centers.

15:40 Michael calls Eurotransplant. H-3 has backed out on the heart, but neither the center nor Eurotransplant had let him know. A fourth heart center (H-4) now has the offer.

15:50 We go up to the operating room to change clothes.

In Germany, surgeons decide to accept an organ based on minimal, basic clinical data (see chapter 8). In the United States, on the other hand, I often observed lengthy descriptions of the donor's overall hospital course. Yet coordinators may reinterpret the donor's data for surgeons—that is, omit or emphasize certain aspects, often to persuade the transplanter to accept the organ, occasionally to dissuade a center from taking it (Hogle 1992, 1995b).

Negotiation Work

During my research I saw how day-to-day decisions and activities reflect local accommodations, resistances, and reinterpretations of supposedly universal, standardized medicine. Surgeons make the ultimate decision about accepting offered organs and giving away or keeping organs they have procured themselves, but coordinators play a key role in mediating information and establishing practices at each transplant center.

According to the system of allocation for kidneys, which is based on matching tissue types (the HLA histocompatibility complex), several rules should apply. After tissue is typed for its HLA profile, an organ is given to the person who best matches the profile. If a perfect match exists, the organ must go to that recipient, regardless of who is next in line or the fact that a needy recipient lives close to the transplant center procuring the organ. This perfect match is rare, so most networks have a rotation system to allocate organs. In the United States an incentive arrangement encourages the procuring OPO to give an organ away to the patient or center next up in the rotation, who is likely to be in another center. At the time of my research among German transplant centers, however, if the kidney had at least two matches of the six antigens, the transplant center that acquired the organ was allowed to keep it for its own recipients rather than give it away. The ambiguity of the in-between matches allows for variability in practices.[5]

In my observations in all parts of Germany, practices differed considerably. Some centers adhered strictly to the policy of giving organs away, but many claimed their right to exceptions, known as local donor allowances. According to a respondent in a major heart center, more than 40 percent of hearts procured by the clinic stay within that clinic. Another study claims that some clinics keep as many as 90 percent of kidneys procured (V. Schmidt 1998).

As one might expect, the situation raises concerns about fairness of allocation. Clinics compete intensely for transplant patients and thus lobby for rules that will get them the most organs. A center with more patients on its waiting list will have a better chance of having a good match within its ranks and be able to perform more procedures. Centers are ranked by ET in order of the numbers of procedures they perform. The more active centers rank higher based on the assumption that with more experience the outcomes are likely to be more successful. Consequently, larger transplant programs have a better chance of getting more organs.

The rules have been modified several times by ET committees in past years as interests from large and small clinics have been deliberated. In 1996 the ET kidney allocation system was revised to put more emphasis on waiting times, geographic distance, and other factors (Bernard Cohen, director of Eurotransplant, personal communication, 1995). A complex point system was created to use alongside tissue matching data. Rules differ by country and by organ, using a combination of factors to balance the needs of sickest patients across the entire network while taking into consideration regional priorities.[6]

Organs allocated to transplant centers on a rotation basis are called center-driven organs. To allocate these organs, transplant centers are ranked by a point system based on the number of procedures performed at the center per year as well as the number of organs procured by that center and whether they are kept in the center or contributed to the pool of available organs. Centers with more points have priority for organ allocation from the ET pool. If a center procures and then gives away the organ to another transplant center (whether or not the organ is eventually used), the procuring center receives extra points: this is supposed to encourage the sharing of organs. If the center procures an organ and then keeps it at the center, points are subtracted as a deterrent to transplanters who do not share with other centers. For active centers with large waiting lists, however, the number of procedures keeps them high in the ranking anyway, so it is more profitable to keep organs for in-house patients.

Patient-driven systems favor the sickest patients independent of the center. But it is possible to manipulate the system by nudging patients into more urgent categories, either by recategorizing them as sicker or actually changing their clinical management. For example, heart patients can be put on medications such as catecholamines. Such medication has temporary and superficial beneficial effects but causes damage and side effects that essentially set the patient on a death course. As one coordinator told me, "it can only work for about six weeks—then they're dead—so these patients *become* more urgent" (f.n., October 1993). Some transplanters I interviewed in Germany and other parts of Europe complained that certain German transplant centers abuse the normal system by registering too many patients as "extremely urgent" to acquire even more of the available pool of organs (f.n., November 1993). Such behavior is not unique to Germany. As I saw in the United States, the decision about who is accepted on the recipient list depends on rankings of urgency and nearness to death—categories plastic enough to allow personnel to add or delete names from the list. This form of gaming may include the patient's ability to pay (f.n., September 1992).

Until recently, organ allocation priority in Germany was also partly determined by the length of time the patient had been on the waiting list. This

created discrepancies between East and West Germans. Before reunification, East German patients without party connections were often not listed
for transplant and did not have as much access to first-tier diagnostic or treatment technology, which was centered in Berlin. Even high-ranked officials
had less opportunity for transplant because of lack of capacity in East Germany. In the first few years after unification, East Germans rarely made it
to transplant: even though they made up 80 percent of the new waiting lists
(because they were diagnosed and put on waiting lists in large numbers),
they had not been on the lists as long as West Germans had at the time of
reunification.

Thus, contrary to ET's public rhetoric about a computer that makes all
decisions objectively, organ distribution is in large part decided by surgeons
at transplant centers. Individual surgeons and procurement coordinators are
able to work around regulations for exchange, reinterpreting medical justifications and using informal criteria.[7]

The way in which organ exchange is organized can have important implications. In Germany, a large multicenter study by Opelz and Wujciak
(Opelz 1992) seems to prove that there are significant differences in outcomes based on HLA antigens. Paid for by the DSO, the study not surprisingly recommends institutionalizing a central body to collect and manage
data and therefore exchanges.

Here is where the story gets more interesting. Many researchers now
argue that the HLA system is meaningless in terms of overall outcomes.
As one American surgeon told me, "Hell, we sometimes transplant livers
across *blood* types, so why should tissue antigens make that much more
difference?" (f.n., January 1992). Indeed, in theory, the advent of a new generation of immunosuppressive drugs should make tissue matching moot.
In addition, new chemical preservatives are coming onto the market that
will mask the immunogenetic features of donor cells.[8]

The controversy has sparked heated debate that will have broad implications. Surgeons who claim not to believe in the HLA system as a predic-
tor of graft success justify bypassing the rules altogether and keeping most,
if not all, organs. Transplanting more patients enhances a center's success
in terms of numbers, ranking, and experience. At the same time, more procedures translate into more clinical and personal income because transplan-

tation is extremely profitable.[9] This limits the entry of new centers and the growth of small centers, which in turn affects current health reform efforts. As states begin to ration services and decide where they should be performed, policymakers take into consideration the number of procedures performed at each clinic.

Thus, existing systems in both Europe and the United States are based on scientific theory and biological constraints but are also shaped by economic interests, competition, and local concerns that clash with supposedly global ideas. The tension between matching human tissue characteristics and allocating scarce resources with some sense of justice has created an open space in which practices vary widely. At the same time, by having a system in place with extensive rules, organ procurement and transplantation maintain the appearance of following straightforward, agreed-upon rules based on scientific judgment.

The following case from my field notes (once again using a pseudonym) illustrates the process of negotiation and the many considerations in offering, accepting, and rejecting an organ. I begin at the point after the first round of offers has been made (f.n., March 1994).

20:40 The first heart transplant center (H-1) calls the coordinator to say it can't take the heart after all.

20:41 The first liver transplant center (L-1) accepts the liver. A second heart center (H-2) is contacted by ET but can only accept the heart if it can have the lungs too; surgeons want to do a domino procedure. (For patients needing a lung transplant, it is easier to transplant the heart also because the blood vessels are too complex to separate. The heart-lung recipient's own heart is removed and available for transplantation into a second recipient.)

20:43 Dieter (the coordinator) calls Eurotransplant, saying, "If there is a domino, and an extra heart is left over, it would be nice if you would look for a recipient in [Dieter names a large clinic in this same town]. The procedure would go very quickly that way." (In other words, a team could get to his clinic more quickly and require less coordination than getting a team from another town.) Dieter explains that his request has to do with the political situation in this town—fierce competition because too many clinics are too close together. He calls the large clinic, letting staff know there may be an available heart so they can be ready and can contact Eurotransplant. He explains that his tip helps improve relations between the clinics and doesn't threaten his own clinic's interest, which transplants kidneys, not hearts.

20:50 Dieter calls another clinic in the same town and asks if it can use the whole pancreas. Surgeons answer no, not without kidneys too. (Patients needing a pancreas transplant due to complications from diabetes do better if they receive a kidney as well.) But Dieter wants to keep the kidneys for his own clinic. He says he will give the pancreas away for research (processing as cells). He calls a cell bank, which arranges for pickup.

In this example, the coordinator worked at making the process more efficient and reducing the waste of valuable resources. So much for the myth that the Eurotransplant computer makes all decisions without human intervention. The role of the coordinator in mediating choices, interpreting data, and facilitating the procedure cannot be underestimated.

Procuring Tissue

Despite increasing regulation and pressure to standardize transnational collection and exchange procedures, tissue is procured in an ad hoc way, particularly in Germany. This indicates not only difficulties in organization but in incentives to procure as well. In most countries, including Germany, tissues are procured either in surgery (immediately after organs for transplant are removed) or in pathology (the hospital morgue). For material removed from brain-dead donors, it is not absolutely necessary for all tissues to be procured under sterile conditions in the operating room: either clean or sterile technique can be used because the patient need not be protected from infection and the tissues are further processed in antibiotic solutions or otherwise treated to decrease microbial content before implanting into a recipient. Thus, removal procedures often occur at a more convenient time and pace—and more inexpensively—in the morgue.

Materials may also be removed during autopsy on patients who have died in the hospital. Pathologists or their assistants remove and store tissues, ship them to banks, or give them to pharmaceutical firms (see chapter 5).

Even when tissue is procured in surgery, an entirely separate team from organ procurement or transplant personnel arrives to acquire the tissues. Often different individuals remove each type of tissue. For example, corneas or entire eyeballs are removed by ophthalmologists, pathologists, or technicians either from the clinic where they will be used or from BioImplant Services. Skin and bone are taken by pathology assistants, technicians, or trauma physicians. Procurers have different skill levels and training, use different protocols, collect different types of data, have different interests, and are responsible to different groups. The infrastructure is also quite different: informal and loosely organized, varying in form and type of participants depending on where and how the materials will be located before final use.

Corneas are evaluated and banked. Skin is sectioned into standard sizes, treated with glycerol, and cryopreserved unless used immediately. Bone is cleaned, cut into a variety of sizes and shapes or processed into powder or gel, and sometimes sterilized before being cryopreserved. The shelf life for most tissue is up to several months (or years for cryopreserved bone components); thus, they can be stored and distributed on demand throughout Europe (Flye 1995).

For heart valves, the entire heart is removed in surgery and sent to a lab or shipped to a bank where technicians remove, inspect, test, and process the valves. Valves may be recovered from hearts discarded from transplant recipients, hearts intended for transplant but not used, or hearts removed from other patients who die in the hospital.

As I have mentioned, tissues are rarely procured in Germany. While this has much to do with cultural meanings of certain body parts and the public's unwillingness to donate tissue, several other factors also limit tissue procurement in Germany. In particular, the lack of coherent organizational structure and other infrastructural elements help explain why efforts are not more coordinated. But there is also evidence of local resistance to and reinterpretation of tissue procurement.

In German medical culture, the attending hospital physician is expected to approach families for donation rather than physicians not associated with the patient (those needing tissue, transplant surgeons, and so on). Yet through their unwillingness to contact families, attending physicians show considerable uncertainty about organ and tissue donation. One survey showed that 45 percent of physicians considered the request for tissues emotionally disturbing and did not want to approach families; 7 percent re-fused outright when directly requested to approach the family (Schütt, Smit, and Duncker 1995).

Promotion and education campaigns among hospital workers to increase tissue donation began to pay off when physicians and nurses increased their referrals to BIS by 1992–93. Nevertheless, referrals from pathology assistants and coordinators dropped sharply between 1991 and 1994 (BioImplant Services 1992, 1993, 1994a). Undoubtedly, this drop is related to the widely publicized scandals about pathology assistants removing cadaver materials for profit (see chapter 5).

During my research, I noted that coordinators were not only reluctant to request permission for tissue donation but even less inclined to arrange for procurement. In the United States, a required consent form explicitly lists each body part to be removed. The German form, however, does not. According to one respondent, coordinators and physicians in Germany frequently include tissues in their mental list of organs:

> Naturally, you have to ask concretely if they will agree to donation without any restrictions. If they ask, "Which organs would be taken?" then one must very clearly say which ones. I say, "Heart, lungs, pancreas, liver, kidneys, and tissue." Tissue I don't explain any further. If they ask, "What is tissue?" then I say, "Bone chips." But what we never take here is skin. (f.n., March 1994)

When I asked organ procurement personnel about their resistance to requesting tissues, they responded consistently that to procure tissues would bring down the entire enterprise. They felt that the public—as well as hospital staff—would object so strongly to procuring such material that relatives would donate nothing at all rather than risk having the body defaced. Moreover, hospital staff would become negative about any material procurement because it would be too disturbing. The following comments notes were typical:

> "Organ donation is like carrying an egg in the hand. You can't let anything disturb it, or it will all go in the air and get broken [makes motion with his hand as if dropping the egg]." (northeastern coordinator, f.n., July 1994)

"Tissues? No, no. It is too much for the staff [the surgical nurses] to bear. We would have a problem with them cooperating." (central western coordinator, f.n., December 1993)

Skin and bone are almost never procured in Germany. Skin in particular seems to be a touchy issue, as the following typical comments show:

"Well, sometimes we take corneas or, rather, get someone to come and take corneas. But skin—no way. It's too much." (northwestern coordinator, f.n., February 1994)

"We take no skin. A hospital should not be burdened in such a way." (southern coordinator, f.n., September 1995)

"I won't ask for tissue. Corneas and valves are no problem. But I won't ask for bones or skin. The people who want this should take care of it themselves and let us take care of organs" (southwestern coordinator, f.n., August 1994)

These were highly sensitive issues, often provoking strong responses. Many respondents tried to avoid answering or otherwise displayed discomfort with the topic:

Coordinator: Sometimes there is a request for corneas, but we don't collect skin.

LH: Why not skin?

Coordinator: We don't need it.

LH: You mean there are no burn cases here? No reconstructive plastic surgery?

Coordinator: Perhaps. But they can order it from a bank in the Netherlands or someplace if they need it.

LH: So where do banks get their skin?

Coordinator: Some other country. . . . Certainly not in Germany.

LH: Yes, but why not Germany?

Coordinator: Well, I think it's just too. . . . *We just don't do it here, that's it!* Why do you want to know about these other things? I don't know anything about these. . . . I get organs. That's hard enough! (f.n., March 1994)

In truth, tissue procurement *is* visually disturbing, but no more so than other types of orthopedic surgery, procedures in which the eye is removed, or when skin is removed from a live patient for self-grafting. Besides, as I have mentioned, these materials can be removed in the morgue by personnel accustomed to removing parts in autopsy.

There are several explanations for why tissue removal is considered disturbing. First, the body is no longer on a respirator, hooked up to monitors, or receiving fluids or blood. It is more distinctly a dead body, and dealing with dead bodies evokes a new set of responses (see, for example, Hogle 1993, 1995c). Moreover, materials are usually not being removed for a specific, identified patient (as in organ transplantation) but stored for eventual general use. Tissue donation is rarely publicized or promoted. Some respondents felt that tissue procurement receives less attention because tissues are usually used for life-improving rather than life-saving illnesses. Still, these explanations are insufficient to explain such extreme reactions.

I believe part of the issue relates to the low-status nature of such work, which is associated with handling dead bodies. Workers who handle the dead—including pathologists but especially nonphysicians—are at the bottom of the medical hierarchy in many western societies (cf. Mitford 1963, *Der Spiegel* 1993a). Judging by how coordinators described their work, I believe they want to associate with higher-order medical work that entails clinical and managerial decision making.

An additional reason for why tissues, particularly skin, may be especially problematic in Germany has to do with rules of formality in everyday life. Touching or handling bodies and too-close physical nearness are taboo in Germany, indicating a lack of respect for the other person. One northern coordinator told me, "To come too close to another person physically disturbs a boundary" (f.n., July 1994). Some Germans with whom I spoke consider the use of IVs and catheters and the extensive touching that takes place in the intensive care unit, especially when a patient is close to death, to be an extreme form of invasion. This notion of invasion applies to handling bodies both before and after death has been proclaimed. It takes a literal form in the case of removing the outer boundary of the body. As one coordinator explained, "skin is too close—too personal" (f.n., December 1993).[10]

Most disturbing, however, are lingering images of skin from concentration camp victims. As I discussed in chapter 3, skin was used for lampshades, book covers, and other decorative items; and many other body products were recycled for a variety of purposes.

Despite the high international value placed on tissue as a finished good on the world market, Germans expend very little effort toward procuring these materials or building an infrastructure that would establish routines for procurement. At the same time, the absence of clear structures and rules allows a private, informal, internal system to proceed that does not require a public face. Materials are acquired through personal contacts or ad hoc arrangements that allow far greater flexibility with fewer controls.

Eight

Converting Human Materials into Therapeutic Tools

U ntil recently, anthropologists of biomedicine took the technical details of medical work at face value. "The investigator stood with his or her back to the heart of medicine and studied the 'social phenomena' surrounding it" (Casper and Berg 1995: 397). This assumption contributed to a deterministic view of science and technology as having an impact *on* the body. I see this process as more interactive. There is a sense in which the objects of medical work themselves constrain theories, tools, work arrangements, scientists, and medical practitioners.[1] In this chapter, I detail the routine, hands-on activities involved in managing the technical and cultural constraints of human materials. At this level of everyday practice, cultural meanings of the body exist amid interactions of particular social, political, economic, and historical contexts.

As previous chapters have shown, infrastructure, organizational aspects, legal presumptions, division of labor, and other work arrangements affect practice. But these arrangements and structures are also shaped by the nature of the tasks necessary to deal with human biological substances. The physical characteristics of the material create a number of constraints. Organs and tissues, after all, are organic, perishable materials. They require a number of chemical and mechanical technologies not only to enable retrieval but to make them useful to practitioners, researchers, and patients. In the process of managing physical characteristics and converting substances into therapeutic tools, the materials are changed physiologically and structurally, becoming part of the technology. That is, physiological functions and cellular structure can be modified to produce desired effects. These transmutations further challenge the categories of human and nonhuman, nature and culture, animate and inanimate previously thought to be straightforward.

Technical restrictions and requirements play a key role in the transformation of medical practices. The material practices of converting body parts into technological tools do more than control the physical characteristics of the tissue. They also deal with the ambiguity that arises around bodies in this new state of being. That is, specific strategies help participants keep the categories of person and thing separate.

Material practices, however, are not universal. On the contrary, they emerge interactively with other elements within both specific local and global contexts. To demonstrate this point, the chapter introduces a number of observations from my previous ethnographic research in the United States as well as German data recorded for this study. Often people assume that the two societies are similar in terms of technological and scientific sophistication and medical practice. The U.S. data, however, show enormous differences in approach, attitudes, and assignment and generation of resources. American practices reveal the locus of activities as the intensive care station and reflect the intensive nature of work that occurs before the removal procedure. In contrast, the most intensive German activities are focused in the operating room, as I discuss in chapter 9. In no case should the reader consider the U.S. data as starting points or norms; they merely illustrate differences.

The chapter is divided into three main sections. I begin by identifying the source of the materials (who—or whose body—is considered to be eligible as a donor) and describe activities involved in transforming a braindead patient into a source of valuable human materials. My point here is that this transformation must be accomplished without appearing to violate bodily integrity or disturb the dead. The next two sections trace the actual practices involved in the conversion of materials into usable therapeutic tools. The first section uses secondary data to describe standard universal practices and includes data from my extensive observations in the United States. Finally, I describe specific practices observed in Germany.

Obtaining Materials without Violating the Person

The conversion of a brain-dead person's body into a usable source of therapeutic tools is the stage at which concerns about inviolability of the body and personhood collide with issues of technological progress and medical authority. How exactly does one obtain and use organs and tissues from dead humans without violating laws, customs, and other protections of bodily integrity? What makes it possible to proceed while claiming not to be disturbing the dead?

The designation of brain death allows a suspension of time during which biomedical experts reconfigure both cultural and biological processes. Creating this ambiguous state of being also requires a number of apparently contradictory practices in dealing with the body. New mechanisms must be created that allow participants to see the human body as existing in a different state. This involves a progressive transformation in status over time and in different spaces.

In my observations in the United States, I noted that the potential donor had a distinct identity as a person up to the time doctors determined that he was probably brain dead and thus a potential organ donor. From this point, there was a continual shift through the process of determining eligibility and the right to use bodily materials up to the time of procurement itself. As soon as brain death was declared, procurement personnel dropped any reference to the person as a patient and ceased using the patient's name. He was thereafter referred to by cause of death, age, or hospital location or simply as the donor; for example, a brain-dead patient may be called "the twenty-four-year-old drive-by shooting at General Hospital" (Hogle 1992).

This is one of several techniques used early in the process to remove the person from the scene—a shift necessary to manage the problem of respecting human boundaries. Compare abortion, in which it is possible to abort a thing but not a person. Similarly, it is possible to procure and use material resources but not a person's remains.[2]

Identifying and Selecting Donors

Which bodies are candidates for the procurement of what organs? Specific criteria predetermined by transplant specialists screen out bodies with tissue that might represent a risk for recipients. Criteria for procurement include absence of HIV, no cancer within the past five years (this varies by type of cancer), no active infection or other condition that might create problems in the recipient (for example, diabetic patients may have kidney damage so are not eligible to donate kidneys), and age (upper and lower limits vary by organ).

As the gap between the number of donors and the increasing number of waiting patients grows, the criteria for selecting donors are relaxed. For example, raising the upper age limit and accepting organs from less healthy donors are ways to increase the pool of eligible donors.[3] In Germany, the median age of donors has increased by eight years since 1990 (Deutsches Stiftung für Organspende 1994). A similar trend exists in the United States, where the number of donors over age fifty increased from 11.7 percent in 1988 to 22.6 percent in 1994. Although organs from less healthy or older donors represent greater risk and potentially poorer function in recipients, the surgeons I interviewed justified their use because of the ready availability of technological intervention: "Even if we take hearts from sixty- or sixty-five-year-olds, we can always do a balloon catheterization later" (f.n., January 1994).

About 40 percent of cadaver donors in Germany become brain dead through head trauma (accidents); the rest have cerebral vascular events or other nontrauma brain damage (Deutsches Stiftung für Organspende 1994). The proportion of trauma victims in the United States is somewhat higher. In the American organ procurement organization I studied, about 50 percent of referred potential donors were victims of violence, motor vehicle accidents, other kinds of accidents, or suicides involving head trauma. In 1994, for the United States as a whole, 49.6 percent were motor vehicle accidents, gunshot or stab wounds, or head traumas. This figure decreased from 59.2 percent in 1988 (United Network for Organ Sharing 1994: 14). The implementation of helmet laws and the proportion of older donors (who tend to die of cerebral bleeding rather than trauma) explain the change in proportions.

It was clear from my observations and interviews that donors in Germany are almost never nonethnic Germans. When I asked why, coordinators explained only that other religions would not permit donation. Assuming that nonethnic Germans (primarily Turks, Africans, and Vietnamese) would object on these grounds, coordinators simply do not approach families for permission. Nor do they take materials without permission. Because there are no records on reasons for not donating or on the potential donor's religion or ethnicity, I could not pursue this question much further. When I pressed, respondents indicated that there might be incompatibility problems related to genetics, which many referred to as "racial factors." Nevertheless, organs and tissues from other countries are accepted for use in German patients. These usually come from Eurotransplant member countries, primarily the Netherlands and Austria, but occasionally Scandinavia.[4]

While the practice of not requesting donation from foreigners was common in western Germany, it was written policy in the east. On my first visit to East German clinics in 1992, I saw instruction sheets and signs on the wall listing factors that would rule out a potential donor. In addition to the usual clinical criteria, *Ausländer* (foreigner) was listed. The reason they gave at the time (and when I asked again in 1994, although the signs were gone) was that there were too many bureaucratic problems with foreign governments to get approval to remove organs from foreigners. Although this argument would apply to visitors from other countries, the criteria were also applied to resident nonethnic Germans, mostly guest workers from Vietnam and eastern Europe. Respondents had no answer for why foreign residents did not fall under the Widerspruchslösung, the East German presumed consent law.

This policy is also curious in light of the fact that several transplant centers are currently making arrangements with eastern European hospitals to train physicians in transplant medicine in exchange for the right to acquire organs there. In future research it would be interesting to learn more about perceptions of crossing ethnic and national boundaries in transplantation—for example, German recipients' opinions about receiving nonethnic German organs. More intriguing would be to explore conceptions of ethnicity as they are tied to physical characteristics of tissue, in terms of either perceived differences in function or immune reaction. Theories about tissue antigen matching and its application to ethnic groups are consequential, particularly in societies with considerable ethnic diversity. How this information is translated into medical knowledge and practice has tremendous implications for policy, organization, allocation of human materials, and evolving technologies.

Materials Source into Therapeutic Tools: Practices in the United States

Once the donor is deemed eligible, she is characterized through information collected about both the body and the person. At this point in the process, practices in the United States and Germany begin to diverge.

Knowing the Person, Knowing the Body

In the United States, I noted an extraordinary amount of activity related to knowing the donor. That is, workers spent a great deal of time and effort obtaining information about both the biological being (the physiological and anatomical status of the body and its organs) and the person (the lived experiential being) who had occupied this body. Data were extracted from the body using numerous diagnostic tools that gave information about the current physiological status of organs and functions. At the same time, workers collected extensive information about the behavior, lifestyle, and social situation of the person from relatives and medical records. This information was intended to reveal the person's stewardship over her body: the way in which she used the body she occupied. The information was combined and differentially used as a screening tool to identify which donors—and which bodies—were desirable candidates. When screened and filtered, the information established which organs and tissues had value as potential therapeutic tools and which should be eliminated from consideration because of perceived risks to the recipient or less perceived value.

Such information was recorded on a standardized form called the donor tracking tool. The clinical progress of the donor during the hospital stay was also tracked on the form: for example, it documented incidents such as cardiac arrest or a too-high level of medication that could cause tissue damage, along with the body's stability and responses over time. The information was used to predict the quality and functionality of the body and its components. Using codes and categories established by UNOS, workers recorded information about cause of death (such as asphyxiation, cerebral hemorrhage, or trauma), circumstances of death (shooting, motor vehicle accident), demographic information (sex, age, occupation, ethnicity), family status, religion, occupation, and other information in addition to clinical data. In 1992, at the beginning of my U.S. fieldwork, the four-page form primarily tracked the clinical management phase. Within seven months it had expanded to sixteen pages and contained almost one thousand data points.

Data from the donor were encoded and restructured into categories. A great deal of information from these donor tracking tools had no immediate application but was collected for possible future studies. Since the way in which data are collected is relatively standardized among U.S. organ procurement organizations, it is possible for research groups, private firms, government agencies, and others to acquire the data for their own purposes. This is a classic example of the way in which information becomes controlled and packaged while becoming less available to previous owners (Poster 1990). Analysts and medical professionals centralize information, which then becomes a commodity itself, available for sale to privileged others. In this way, information management is a byproduct of human materials technology, further influencing work and social arrangements.

The medical history section of the donor tracking tool was expanded to identify a variety of possible contraindications for donation. Changes included the straightforward registration of incidences of hepatitis, cancer, diabetes, active intravenous drug use, heart disease, and other chronic diseases that affect transplantable organs and tissues. The form also listed social conditions that could signal the presence of dangerous tissue without directly indicating disease: traveling outside the United States, residence in a long-term care facility, and tattoos.[5]

Additionally, a section was added for social history, including "Has the deceased ever had sex with a male who has ever had sex with another male?" and "Has the deceased ever been in jail?" Medical and social histories were often combined, as in a section used to describe the events leading up to the death, which contained notes such as "practiced Satanism," "$5,000 found in car," "estranged from family," "parents divorced at age 17," "the mom had alcohol at the hospital," and numerous other comments that had little or nothing to do with the medical condition of the body or the cause of death. Lengthy narratives were constructed and retold about the donor's life history and circumstances, family relationships (including who visited at the hospital and how they behaved), and the donor's personality ("generous," "religious," "always in trouble") (f.n., February 1992). All these "data" were combined with medical data to present a picture of a good or a bad donor. That is, in the United States, behavioral attributes and moral status played a central role in determining both donor eligibility and organ quality. The information constructed a story not only about the nature and worth of the bodily materials but also the worth of the person as a potential donor. Significantly, however, eligibility was not necessarily tied to actual use of certain bodies as donors. Rather, there were a number of cases in which the quality of the donation outweighed the quality of the donor in deciding which donors to use (Hogle 1995b).

Knowledge about the user of the body—and thus the presumed uses of the body during the potential donor's lifetime—was combined with knowledge about the physiological status of specific organs at the time of death. Diagnostic tests and clinical measurements were performed as frequently as every two hours. The cadavers underwent echocardiograms and even CAT scans and cardiac catheterizations in an attempt to obtain a more accurate picture of organ function and predict whether the organ would make a successful graft. Coordinators reported this information to the surgeons who had been offered organs, who then decided to accept or reject them based largely on the combined physiological, clinical, and social history data.

It was not unusual to move the cadaver to another hospital where more high-tech equipment was available to diagnose its condition. In an age of increasing managed care and cost controls, the expense and labor involved were considerable. Such intense activity is possible only within highly developed infrastructures; broad social and political acceptance; and cooperation from payers, the public, hospital personnel, and donors' families.

Extraordinary effort and expense, then, were spent in imaging and characterizing targeted organs. This has the effect of removing the body as a whole from view in much the same way that modern imaging technologies have constructed the fetus as a separate entity from the mother (Casper 1994, 1998, Hartouni 1991). The body is reimagined as a container and life support system for the targeted organs.

The focus on organs rather than the body as a whole intensified in later phases of the process. As the time for removing materials neared, workers rarely referred to the body or person at all. Rather, they made references to the specific materials to be removed. "What's the progress on the heart at General Hospital?" or "Who's covering the kidneys at Valley Hospital?" were common statements. At this point, they also dropped descriptions of the circumstances or cause of death as well as other social information critical to donor selection (Hogle 1995b).

Another type of intimate knowledge develops simply through handling and working with the body in the process of transforming the patient into a donor. For American coordinators, these activities were intense. Coordinators tended to spend a great deal of time in the room with the donor rather than in office spaces. Most activity was related to adjusting the technology: observing monitor changes, going over data, changing medications and fluids, inserting new arterial lines, moving limbs to better accommodate lines or enhance blood pressure, and removing blood for testing. Coordinators helped nursing staff by suctioning the lungs and performing a variety of other body maintenance activities (Hogle 1992, 1995b). Because of the intensity of work, there was often a nursing staff-to-patient ratio of two to one.

Ironically, even with these constant manipulations, the body as a patient's body seemed to disappear. Visually, the body was barely evident under the forest of equipment. It was usually completely covered with an electronic warmer and connected to a ventilator, monitors, and IV solution pumps. The head was also usually covered, especially if there had been substantial trauma to the head or face. Two to four catheters were inserted into veins and arteries so that chemicals could be injected and blood withdrawn for testing as well as to monitor blood pressure.[6]

Donors' bodies were represented on the donor tracking tool (see figure 8.1). Injuries to the body, scar tissue, and physical anomalies were marked on the diagram, representing the body in realistic detail. The diagram normalized the donor as a mesomorphic male (without genitalia) but otherwise indicated facial features, hair, and musculature.

Thus, by collecting personal and bodily information, manipulating the body, and re-creating the person and her body on paper, the donor is *known*. The information procured and the knowledge constructed is then displaced into another material form. In a sense, what remains is an identity without a body. Through representations created by imaging technologies, the donor becomes transparent and the parts more visible. The body as a whole entity disappears and is disseminated, transmuted into two-dimensional form. Ultimately, it is literally fragmented and distributed. But the person lives on in the data. Essentially, he is transferred from the biological body and reinscribed into representational data, reimagined as a "generous per-

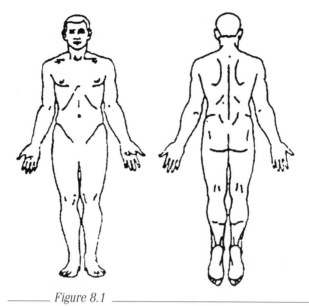

———— *Figure 8.1* ————————————————————
Representation of Donor Bodies, United States

son who would have wanted to help someone else" or a "troubled youth whose wasted life can be redeemed by helping others."[7]

Transferring or displacing the person while focusing on targeted body parts is one strategy used to deal with the ambiguities of the living cadaver while allowing access to bodily materials. At the same time, narratives about and reconstructions of the donor act as a commemoration and gesture of respect for the dead.

Managing the Materials

He who calibrates, controls.
(Bruno Latour, *Science in Action* [1987])

In addition to cultural constraints related to personhood, workers must deal with technical constraints associated with the physical character-istics of the body and its tissues. The brain-dead body is kept in the intensive care unit, where it can be closely monitored until procurement. In the United States, donors are usually kept in a separate room. American transplant professionals call activities from brain death to procurement "donor management." Donor management in the United States can begin long before brain death is officially diagnosed and can last for several days while logistics (including family matters) are worked out (Hogle 1992).[8]

Management of the donor is necessary because of the many physiological changes that take place when the brain ceases to function. Blood begins to coagulate in the distal limbs, and the vascular system collapses. Cell walls become rigid, changing their permeability to fluids and molecules. Cardiac arrhythmias and arrests can occur. A number of conditions are common in brain-dead patients, such as diabetes insipidus, in which the hypothalamus cannot control fluids. In effect, the body is trying to die.

The brain-dead "patient," then, creates a new set of clinical and cultural dilemmas. Certain physiological conditions require that maintenance and resuscitation techniques normally used on living patients are used on the donor's "dead" body.[9] Such measures confuse the usual understandings of "patient care" and the role of care providers. For example, routine cardiopulmonary resuscitation protocols (electric shock, cardiac massage, and so on) may be used to restart an arrested heart in the cadaver. The body is no longer able to regulate its own functions, so a number of mechanical and chemical technologies substitute for normal functions. Breathing, blood pressure, temperature control, fluid and electrolyte balance, and hormone production must be managed externally. The lungs, brachia, and stomach must be suctioned routinely to remove excess fluids. The body is hormonally stimulated to create urine. In major trauma cases, many units of blood have to be replaced (cf. Wijnen and van der Linden 1991).

In the intensive donor management I observed in the United States, massive amounts of fluids, blood (if the patient sustained major traumatic injuries), and pharmaceutical agents were circulated through the body to replace fluid volume and keep physiological systems in balance. Glucose was given to stimulate ATP production and store glycogen to produce and store metabolic energy for better post-transplant function. Antibiotics were administered as a prophylaxis against infection. Colloids and crystalloids, dopamine, mannitol, Lasix, electrolyte products, fibrin, and other chemicals were used to balance fluid and body chemistry because the brain could no longer perform these functions (Kaufman 1986; Novitzky, Cooper, and Reichert 1987; Soifer and Gelb 1989). Alpha blockers counteracted the release of catecholamines that occurred immediately after brain ischemia or if the heart arrested to prevent heart tissue damage. Prostaglandins prevented platelet aggregation, which typically occurs when the vasculature collapses. Close monitoring was necessary to keep these chemicals in balance and to prevent the administration of a chemical given to correct one problem from adversely affecting other physiological systems.

Such interventions keep the body system as a whole functioning while maintaining individual organs and tissues in viable condition for explantation. To control conditions and eliminate variations in practices, workers in the United States (and increasingly in Europe) use standardized protocols for clinically managing donors (de Jong and Kranenburg 1995; see also Hogle 1995b). The primary goal of these treatments is to produce "prime-quality organs," as one respondent told me (f.n., May 1992). Yet some of these standard protocols and chemicals are used in nonstandard ways. While some of the procedures are routine intensive care protocols designed for living (or less brain-injured) patients, others are designed to work in ways that could injure a live patient. For example, to prevent brain swelling and further damage to brain tissue, workers would normally withhold fluids from a brain-injured patient expected to live. In a donor, however, workers want to keep tissues hydrated but do not try to retard or prevent further damage. According to one coordinator leading a training session, "you want to make the patient finish his [brain] herniation" (f.n., April 1992). Occasionally this goal means that protocols conflict. For example, mannitol (a diuretic given to regulate fluids) is an impermeate for kidneys but not for livers; that is, although it does not cause fluid to enter kidney cells, it does cause fluid to enter liver cells, creating swelling. Similarly, some vasopressors such as dopamine and norepinephrine sustain blood pressure but impair liver metabolism. In this way, organs—and transplant teams—are sometimes pitted against each other in a bizarre survival of the fittest. These conflicts have to be negotiated by the coordinator, the various transplant teams that will use each organ, and occasionally the attending physician.

The donor management phase is crucial to both the maintenance and preservation of organs. The term *preservation* once referred to the phase in which the organ is removed and preserved in a special fluid before being implanted in the recipient. Increasingly, however, it refers to the period of donor management before the organs are removed. Workers are putting more effort into preparing materials while they are still in the body rather than simply performing preventive measures in the recipient.

Reordering Nature

New pharmaceutical agents designed specifically for use in brain-dead potential donors go beyond simple maintenance. These chemicals preserve cell integrity, inhibit certain functions while enhancing others, and capture metabolic byproducts that cause tissue necrosis. These agents include free oxygen radical scavengers such as allopurinol and verapamil, which remove metabolic byproducts that cause damage when released.[10] Further, some compounds are being tested that will change cellular characteristics to prevent subsequent reaction in the recipient's body (Motoyama et al. 1995). Through these interventions, organs and tissues become more like universal parts—like off-the-shelf reagents. At the same time, they are reconstructed to make them "more real": arguably more like a kidney than a "natural" kidney. Through technological augmentation, they become more functional, less vulnerable and longer-lasting—suitable for use in a variety of bodies.

These approaches could be called donor enhancement. Through them, the body becomes new type of human-technology composite—what I call elsewhere a *donor-cyborg* (Hogle 1995c). The nature of the entire body, even down to individual cells, is changed; conditions incompatible with life for the body in which they exist will nevertheless artificially extend life for another body. This is a perfect example of Marilyn Strathern's (1992) claim that we can no longer refer to technology and nature as distinct domains that can function as metaphors for each other. This is how technology helps life to work.

One effect of using enhancement technologies is that they allow for more time and flexibility in the process. Rather than simply matching a suitable donor with a recipient, workers can optimize recipient selection. They also allow the collection of even more data. The procurement procedure can be organized more efficiently for the transplanters and procurers: for example, the time between declaration of legal death and removal of materials can be altered to suit the needs of procurers and recipients. In the process, however, the death process is reordered. Usual rituals, behaviors, and grieving patterns give way to new ones devised for this unique situation.

Materials Sources into Therapeutic Tools: Practices in Germany

In general, my observations of donor management were typical of descriptions in international clinical literature and comments I heard from surgeons and coordinators around Europe. What differed in Germany was the extent to which diagnostic and preservation technologies were employed, the aggressiveness with which potential donors were pursued, and the extensive amount of personal and social information collected about potential donors. The way in which information was interpreted and used also differed from my experience in the United States. Both in 1992 and then again in 1993 through 1994, I noted that German workers followed standard protocols for very basic donor intensive care maintenance, but their patterns of handling the body, data collection and use, pacing, and location were strikingly different. I am not implying, however, that standardized protocols followed in other countries were not followed in Germany. Interpretations, modifications, and resistances are made locally wherever they are applied.

Bodies, Persons, and Identities

In Germany there is no imagined history of the donor pieced together from narratives and very little official history: German coordinators record only name, sex, age, weight, size, and cause of death. Minimal, basic clinical data were taken once or perhaps twice a day rather than every two to four hours, as in the United States. The same screening criteria apply (HIV status, evidence of cancer or other disease, and so on), but coordinators asked for little or no information about the social status of the individual, behavioral attributes, or other personal information. Several times I observed that coordinators had to be reminded of the age or even the gender of the donor, and they knew few details about the circumstances of death.

I routinely asked coordinators to recall and describe a particular case step by step. A few described specific cases, usually ones with which they had a sense of personal connection: for example, if the donor was the same age and sex as their own child or had a condition that their own relative had died from. Most, however, described a generalized composite case, using the third person to discuss activities. Their descriptions usually focused on conflict with physicians in the donor hospital or the transplant clinic or on activities in the operating room.

German coordinators used no standardized form for data collection. Some, but not all, forms included a representation of the individual's body (see figure 8.2). In contrast to the representation of the donor on the U.S. form, the body shown here is nothing more than a schematic diagram of shapes upon which injuries are roughly represented. It has no facial features, and the limbs and body are distorted or missing. Very little identifies the figure as human.

Workers did use echocardiograms and X rays but rarely employed other imaging technologies that visualized organs. When such technologies were used, they did not seem to be the deciding factor in accepting or rejecting organ offers.

Ready-Made Materials

In stark contrast to the United States, coordinators in Germany spend little time on the clinical management of donors. The coordinator can make suggestions to intensive care staff about donor management; and if he is a physician, these suggestions are more likely to be followed. But while coordinators described donor management as one of their duties, many intensive care nurses disagreed. They said that any administration of pharmaceuticals is performed by nursing staff under the supervision of the intensive care physician—who is only occasionally present.

Coordinators seldom entered the donor's room. They also rarely touched the body, and then only to check for swelling or injury sites, look for evidence of intracavity fluid, or occasionally help insert a cannula.[11] If the donor was in the hospital where the coordinator was based, he was more involved in actual management. Still, the intense monitoring, testing, and chemical injection I saw in the United States were not matched in Germany, despite the availability of such pharmaceuticals and technologies.

Western German physicians told me that eastern physicians tend to do more of this donor handling work, which in the west is done by the nursing staff. I did not observe enough difference to support these assertions but found it to be an interesting perception. It implied that direct contact with the patient was lower-status work but also represented more solidarity with other types of workers. Coordinators, surgeons, and nurses in the east constantly described a sense of teamwork and interchangeability of roles in their clinical work before reunification.

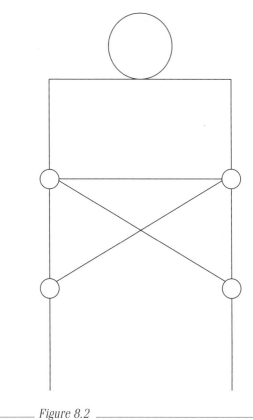

———— *Figure 8.2* ————
Representation of Donor Bodies, Germany

The following field notes from two procurements describe some of my observations:

We go into the unit only one time where the donor is with two other patients and one empty bed. We are asked [by the intensive care nurse] to put on extra gowns while in the room.[12] We stay only briefly. [The coordinator] doesn't approach the body, doesn't check monitors or lines. I go in later by myself, but there are no nurses around to question. [The coordinator] enters the room only once in three and a half hours. (f.n., July 1994)

Not until an hour after we arrive do we go into the donor's room. He is in a small room with a living elderly woman. [The coordinator] visually looks over his chest and quickly probes the body to feel the size of the liver. Otherwise he does not check the body. (This is not a traumatic injury case.) We never reenter the room. (f.n., February 1994)

These patterns held true for both physician and nonphysician coordinators. They stayed near the phone in the intensive care unit's office, often minimizing their presence as much as possible, especially if the hospital physicians or nursing staff were negative or ambivalent toward organ donation (which is fairly common in Germany).

Donors were often kept in rooms with living patients, partly because intensive care space was at a premium. Since beds were in demand for living patients, a donor rarely had a private room. (This space issue applied to the United States as well, although donors were still kept separate in each case I observed there.) Both men and women were naked and left uncovered from the waist up. In fact, far more of the body was visible than was the case in the United States. According to one example in my field notes, "everything looks like the normal ICU routine. Like other donors I have seen, though, she is uncovered, nothing on her head, no warmers, minimal lines" (f.n., August 1994). In contrast, American donors are kept in hospital gowns, or their bodies are covered with sheets or towels. Genitalia and faces in particular are hidden from view. Among American workers, exposing certain body parts was considered improper. One wonders, however, if the affront was to the deceased or to the staff caring for her. In Germany the donor's body was more visible, but it was not viewed—rather, not *seen*.

The lack of detailed information about the donor or her life and history creates a situation in which the body is present but the person is absent. In short, in the United States, there is an identity without a body; in Germany there is a body without an identity. Paradoxically, in Germany it is the exterior—the opaque body—that is visualized rather than its parts, which will be inspected directly in great detail "in the hand" but not through their representations (see chapter 9). In both the United States and Germany, the body is handled as though it is different from a patient. But by not making an effort to cover the person and having minimal interaction with the body, Germans have created a strategy for making the body object-like from the outset.

At this point it may be helpful to consider the German treatment of living patients. I went on rounds in the intensive care station at two clinics and observed that physicians stood at some distance from the beds, often held their hands behind their backs, and rarely approached or touched patients except to inspect wounds (and this was usually done visually). In this sense, the distance from dead bodies is not so different from formal distance from the living patient and could even indicate a type of respect, as it would in formal social interaction in Germany.

As I mentioned in chapter 7, many Germans consider IVs and other inserted devices to be violations of the body. Friends and colleagues spoke to me about their parents' deaths—how unnatural it was even to have routine catheters (arterial, venous, or urinary) in the bodies of the dying. Two respondents used the term *Beleidigung* (insult to the dead). Thus, Germans' less intense manipulations of the dead body might be partly explained by ways of thinking about invading bodily boundaries of the living and the dying. But if donor management as prescribed by the international literature supposedly guarantees better outcomes, and if Germany suffers from an organ shortage (making every donor precious), why do German practitioners differ from other countries in their donor management practices?

Found Objects: Natural Objects Naturally Produced

In my observations of German practitioners, I was particularly struck by their eschewal of measures intended to change tissue characteristics. Coordinators consistently told me that such measures made no difference to graft survival or outcomes. Furthermore, they emphasized a preference for keeping donor materials in a more natural state. To be more functional, they said, materials should be *lebensfrisch*—fresh from the living body and thus closer to the animate and natural state. German coordinators tended to refer to donor management procedures as "organ protection therapy": activities meant to maintain a certain state rather than changing or managing the conditions. They suggested that organs can be supported but not improved. In other words, Germans viewed the outcome as depending on the inherent individual characteristics of each organ from each donor.[13] Given these different standards, workers felt little need to perform intensive procedures on the body or to apply a variety of technologies at this point in the process.

In sum, German use of space and treatment of the body in the place where it remains before the actual explantation procedure are different from patterns observed in the United States. Time use also differs: in Germany, 65 percent of explantations occur within eight hours after declaration of brain death. In the United States, prospective testing and placement of donors sometimes begins long before formal brain death is declared, and management can last for several days (Hogle 1992). Eight hours is a very short time span in which to organize the necessary people and materials for either procurement or management.

With less intensive management to stabilize donor bodies and prevent decline in physiological status, Germans need to compress the time as much as possible. At the same time, they must respond to the sensitized environment in which organ procurement takes place. Coordinators work discreetly and quickly, minimizing contact with hospital staff, who are often unsure about or hostile to the enterprise.

These patterns indicate the particular contextual variables in the German setting. The existence of controversy means that participants want to finish the work quickly with a minimum of visibility. It also means that hospital staff may be resistant to the work. Certainly, it means that different participants have different meanings regarding the body and the events. Hierarchical relations in the medical profession affect who makes the decisions and who handles the body. Organizationally, those who are responsible for procuring materials are also directly involved in the implantation of materials into recipients and follow-up with these patients. Explicit identification with the transplantation enterprise makes direct involvement in patient care, declaration of brain death, and early phases of donor management problematic in a setting in which the acceptance and interests of physicians are highly controversial. This is another reason why in Germany the brain-dead patient, once he moves to the status of donor, never becomes a person to the new group of actors who work with him.

Physiological, Technological, and Cultural Interventions

Social theorists have analyzed the ways in which scientists continually negotiate various elements of local settings to make things work.[14] Included among these elements are the work arrangements, scientific theories, tools, and materials necessary for the project. The interaction among these elements constitutes practice. In organ and tissue procurement, the tools and materials are extraordinary, crossing over tidy boundaries of tool, work object, and human being.

Organs and tissues, if they are to be procured for use as tools, must be accessed through an ambiguous body. The brain-dead body is both a protective container for these therapeutic tools and a physical and cultural barrier.[15] The body has been legally and medically defined as dead, but it has not died; the tissues are still living. In this suspended and liminal state, the donor cadaver exists in two cognitively distinct yet interwoven spheres: person and thing. Specific cultural mechanisms have emerged that enable disaggregation of the social person and the biological being in ways that ameliorate these tensions and deal with the ambiguities related to entities that are simultaneously precious human remains, technological artifacts, waste products, and therapeutic tools. Only in this way can changes be made in handling the body at death and new uses allowed for the materials from the body. Access to and use of the biological being must be sanctioned by legal, social, and scientific conventions, just as it was in the eighteenth century, when the bodies of executed prisoners were used as teaching and curative tools.

German media accounts and popular debates often criticize transplant medicine for violating *Totenruhe* (the peace of the dead) and not allowing persons *Frieden zu Sterben* (to die in peace), arguments rarely used in the United States. Because of the history of bodily violation under National Socialism and the invasions of the private sphere under both the Nazis and the Stasi, probing a person's life history as well as touching and entering her body can seem like invasions. Handling and intervening with the body, then, must be minimized both to preserve its classification as a thing and to retain the image that medical professionals are performing a service without appearing to violate the bodies of the dead. Minimizing manipulations and activity around the dead body before organs are removed means less apparent intervention with natural processes, making the controversial aspects of transplant medicine less visible. Organs and tissues are maintained in a natural state meant to sustain the ability to animate and regenerate life in the recipient.

Because there is only minimal contact with the body and little information collected about the donor, German donors never become known as individuals with histories. A donor simply never becomes a person. This is key because in Germany a person cannot be perceived to die in order for someone else to live. Thus, while the organ can "live on," as described in transplant rhetoric, the person must not. Controlling the technical constraints of the tissue proceeds in tandem with controlling the human source. The very fact that something must be done to demarcate persons from materials sources indicates very old, unresolved issues about social and biological transitions at death. The late twentieth-century body does not simply exist as a commodity; the techniques may differ, but the body must be transformed in much the same way as it has in centuries past.

Nine

The Right Therapeutic Tools

The activities of coordinators, surgeons, managers, politicians, and others are central to constructing the meanings surrounding the use of organs and tissues from brain-dead bodies. The fate of the materials also depends on the work of these various participants in negotiating when, where, and in whom organs will be used, as well as the conditions under which participants' decisions are made.

First, protocols, instruments, techniques, and theories are adapted to the extraordinary situation of removing organs and tissues from a so-called "living cadaver." In some ways the body is treated like a living patient undergoing surgery. But other practices belie the assumption of standard surgical practice, indicating instead the ambiguous nature of the surgical object. Second, scientific knowledge is differentially interpreted and applied in various contexts. Knowledge bases with which to evaluate organs for use are woven together differently, and decision making is located at different points in the process. The body itself is involved in knowledge production, both in its symbolic meanings and physiological responses. This has implications for the organization of procurement and distribution locally, nationally, and internationally, as it does for further development of related technologies. Local interpretations and meanings co-evolve with the processes of applying knowledge to create a theory of how to handle human material and adapt techniques and tools.[1]

The Procurement Procedure: Adapting Tools and Techniques to a Living Cadaver

An administrative and political space was articulated
upon a therapeutic space. . . . Out of discipline, a medically useful space was born.
(Michel Foucault, *Discipline and Punish* [1979], 144)

The operating room (OR) is a necessary but contradictory space in the processing of an organ and tissue donor. Procedures and temporal-spacial organization in the operating room are among the most patterned and prescribed in medical care. Normally, this space is reserved for repairing or restructuring, usually for therapeutic purposes. In the case of organ procurement, the space is used for a nonroutine procedure on a nonroutine patient. Different types of administrative and political articulations are made in a space that is intended to be used as a place for therapy. But for organ and tissue replacement, the therapy is not being enacted at this site but at the site where the recipient is being prepared to accept the implant. Transplant professionals, however, depict the organ and tissue recovery procedure as an unfortunate but necessary phase in the therapy itself—the invisible part. Participants know that the operating room is a temporary stop: rather than returning to another space where healing and restoring will continue, this body is sent on to the morgue. As soon as the heart is clamped off and circulation ceases, any debate over whether or not brain death is real death is pointless. In the retrieval of human materials, then, the operating room becomes a site where life and death, therapy and dismemberment dangerously intermingle.

Other uncommon and uncontrolled elements move through this space: nationalities, languages, social statuses, belief systems, laws, and regulations all cross borders to participate here. These interminglings make standardized protocols and universal medical knowledge vulnerable, creating a space for change. Here, the invasion of bodies, identities, and territories is permitted. In such an assemblage, practices are interactive and evolving.

Organ procurement procedures must be performed under sterile conditions, so the body must be moved from intensive care to the OR before a procedure begins. This means that the procedure competes with elective and emergency surgeries (profit-generating procedures) that fill the OR schedule during the day. Since procurement procedures are not scheduled and the host hospital receives only minimal cost coverage, they are usually performed during the night, avoiding peak daytime hours. This may require bringing in on-call employees (scrub nurses and other OR staff) because many smaller hospitals do not staff the operating room overnight. In Germany I often saw a body being brought down to surgery completely covered (head also) as though it was headed for the morgue but being manually ventilated en route to supply oxygen to tissues. This bizarre sight graphically illustrates the fact that the body is being treated as both dead and alive.

My role as observer shifted during this phase. In the OR, everyone is dressed and masked in the same way, and it is difficult to distinguish a surgeon from a visitor. Moreover, everyone becomes more directly involved in the activities; and among those not performing surgery at the table, a type of camaraderie starts when they remove street clothes and don surgical attire. From my field notes:

> There is only one changing room about the size of a supply closet. I wait for the guys to get there and go first. As I undress (very quickly), others come in. I always have a problem finding small-sized clogs and greens [surgical dress], but this is an opportunity to talk with OR staff when I ask for help. This is a different social space—a leveling space for gender and hierarchy, except for the surgeons, of course. We introduce ourselves. [The coordinator] tells me I can use the informal *du* with him instead of *Sie*. At the end, it is the same. [The coordinator] comes in, and we talk while we are dressing. No one seems uncomfortable or prudish about bodies as we would in the United States. (f.n., July 1994)

At this point, people begin filtering into the operating room: first the anesthesiologist and the coordinator, then the OR nurse. The first transplant team to arrive usually begins the opening procedure unless there is an in-house surgeon present. The pace is slow and calm. Preparation and opening of the body must be timed carefully. Often there is a balancing game between when the operating room is available and when explanting teams get there. Teams can be delayed due to weather conditions (they usually fly via helicopter), their own scheduling interests, or uncertainty about whether to accept the organ based on available information.

The body is draped and prepped using sterile routines, just as in other types of surgery. Arms are sometimes extended at right angles to the body to make room for cannulae, drains, IVs, and other necessary equipment. While the body is visible, this "crucifixion pose" is startling; but the body is soon covered for the procedure.[2]

Once the others arrive, there are more physicians and assistants around the table than is usual for routine surgery. The thoracic and abdominal teams consist of one or two surgeons each, surgical assistants, a coordinator, and sometimes a perfusionist from the transplant centers. The host hospital supplies additional surgical assistants and the circulating nurse, who responds to requests for supplies and acts as a factotum. Also present are the coordinator who organized the procurement at the host hospital and occasional observers (besides myself), especially those from university centers. The coordinator, circulator, and observer are in constant motion during the procedure: moving or getting needed equipment, observing the procedure, or simply getting out of the way. Most rooms are small, designed for no more than four or five persons around the patient, but for a procurement it is common to have as many as seventeen people in the room.

Coordinators usually do not participate in the removal of organs and tissues but work around the edges of the room, preparing flush and packing solutions, tracking data, and responding to surgeon requests. They also act as communicators, telephoning data to waiting transplant centers and to Eurotransplant. The primary role of coordinators at this point is to facilitate the work flow and organize timing and tasks—the often invisible "articulation work" of managing multiple simultaneous trajectories (Strauss et al. 1985).

Thus, while the work of coordinators is critical to the procedure, it constitutes a separate sphere of activity. There is often (but not always) a sense of camaraderie among the coordinators from the different transplant clinics and a degree of informality that I did not experience with the surgeons. From my field notes: "When the liver team gets there, its coordinator recognizes me: "Mensch! You're everywhere!" The coordinators on this case all know each other: they are all old-timers. There is much joking around, standing close to each other (me in the middle) and physical touching/bumping—something that would never occur in the office or even other clinical settings" (f.n., October 1994).

During the procedure, the body is covered except for the incision site. While it looks like a passive object, the body still has a type of agency. That is, in addition to the variety of perceptions about links of the body to the human person, the body responds physiologically to its internal and external environments during the explantation procedure. In this way, the nature of the body as an actant constrains the other actants in the way in which they relate to the body as either a technological object or a dead patient (Akrich 1992: 206). For example, as the body responds to the loss of blood and other effects of surgery, support measures and hemodynamic systems must be carefully maintained. More disconcerting are reactions not considered to be characteristics of dead bodies. Spinal reflexes may cause the body to move, as if the body is reacting to the incisions. Blood pressure and respiratory changes have been reported at the moment of incision and during the procedure. Neither reaction is supposed to happen in "dead" bodies, even brain-dead ones, and neither the chemical agents nor the physical actions being carried out explain such reactions in the reported cases (Wetzel et al. 1985, Emmrich 1994c).

The anesthesiologist or anesthetist administers pancuronium or other anesthetic agents to inhibit such reflex neuromuscular activity, but no other anesthetic agents are used. This has raised questions among some OR staff members I talked with in Germany: since no deep-pain control is used, individuals who are unsure or unconvinced about the implications of brain death are concerned that the person may be able to sense pain even if he is incapable of expressing it. Therefore, he may be dying an agonizing death, according to detractors. Neurologists insist that pain response is no longer possible in brain death. Not using additional anesthesia is another way of cognitively placing the body closer to the state of being an organic mass as opposed to a patient in an indeterminate state of animation. This is not to say that it is intentional abuse or lack of respect for the body as much as a way of maintaining perceptual categories of life and death. In any case, both opinions about pain response are theoretical because they are impossible to test. The reflexes and the attempts to control them indicate the interactivity between the donor and the surgical team. Both flinch: the donor's body reacts to unexpected intervention (whether from the injury that caused the brain death or from the surgeon's knife), and the surgeon and the anesthesiologist react to an unanticipated response that you wouldn't expect from an "object." One is an invasion of bodily boundaries, the other an invasion of the boundary between death and life.

When the body is disinfected, positioned, draped, and connected to the appropriate monitors and equipment, the procedure begins. The incision is made midline from the base of the throat to the pubis, and anchoring ligaments and the diaphragm are severed to create a wider than usual separation of the central area. This allows maximum visualization and accessibility to all of the anatomy, even if not all thoracic and abdominal organs will be procured. Large Balfour retractors are used to open a much wider area than is common in most surgical procedures.[3] In one case, a surgeon made an additional transverse incision through the midsection of the body, cutting a giant X. He proceeded to pull the flaps of flesh back and suture them to the trunk of the body. This was an extraordinary move, one I had never seen before (or since), even in autopsy. Both nursing staff and physicians from other teams were extremely uncomfortable about this, commenting about the surgeon and attempting to make jokes that no one laughed at. Afterward, the coordinator in charge apologized profusely for the *Ausschlachtung* (butchery) of the surgeon's method. Even though the living cadaver was considered to be a thing instead of a human person's remains, participants found this treatment of the body repugnant.[4]

Procurement procedures require more adjustment and adaptation of routines and equipment than do other types of surgery. Instruments for normal surgery are usually pregrouped and sterilized as a set specific to certain kinds of surgical procedures. There is no standard instrument set for organ procurement because it is not frequently performed at most hospitals, so a thoracotomy set (for the thorax) and a laparotomy set (for the abdomen) are both used to start with. Since procurement procedures are nonstandard, however, and usually performed during the night, instruments may not be preprocessed and available. Explanting surgeons must improvise: occasionally, autopsy instruments, instruments that are the wrong size, or instruments commonly used for other purposes must be substituted. From my field notes: "There is some discussion because no spreaders are available. The nurses say there isn't another one. Someone retrieves a strange folding spreader, probably from an autopsy set. All act surprised, but they figure out how to adapt it" (f.n., October 1994).

I have also seen instruments used immediately after being sterilized, which almost never occurs in surgery on live patients. Steam-sterilized instruments are far too hot for tissues, and ethylene oxide–sterilized instruments need to be aerated for several hours to prevent toxic gas from entering the surgical site.

These practices illustrate the contingent and nonstandard nature of this extraordinary procedure. Fortunately or unfortunately, contingencies sometimes involve people. Often, there may only be one surgeon available in the middle of the night, particularly in smaller towns. This happened during one observation, with a result familiar to anthropological fieldworkers. From my notes: "The teams are late, and the kidney 'team' is only one surgeon with no one to assist. The surgeon makes the initial incision, then turns to me and asks, 'Do you want to assist in the operation?' I decline. The physician coordinator assists, and one scrub nurse eventually comes to the table" (f.n., July 1994).

Following are excerpts from my notes during another procurement, demonstrating difficulties that may arise once the teams are inside the body:

> 20:48 They are opening an hour late. The coordinator takes down information on all staff in the room. Surgeons from the host hospital begin opening and preparation before heart and liver teams get there.
>
> 21:30 The kidney team surgeon is having difficulty getting the left kidney. He turns his body to face the donor's feet and has his right arm stretched behind him, up past his elbow within the body cavity, pulling and reaching, pushing other structures out of the way. There is more internal damage [due to the accident] than was previously thought, and the liver looks swollen.
>
> 21:45 The liver team calls; they will be a half-hour late. The work is slowed down, and we wait.
>
> 22:30 The heart team arrives. Its coordinator got there before the surgeons. I recognize him, and we begin to talk about routines in his country. Because there are teams from more than one country present, everyone is supposed to communicate in English. But teams are going about their business without much communication. (f.n., October 1994)

In another procedure, the body was opened, organs inspected, and the heart was rejected by the heart team. A team from another transplant center was called to come and take a look at the heart, and the entire procedure was halted until they arrived. The open body cavity was covered with a towel for an hour and twenty minutes. The anesthesiologist stayed by the body, and the rest of us adjourned to the lounge to await the new team's arrival.[5] This meant that the kidney and liver teams had to wait to get their organs, house staff had to stay longer (it was two o'clock in the morning), and the body could have easily become unstable. Because of hard-to-get donors, however, the coordinator decided to try to use the heart. Ultimately, the second team also rejected the heart.

Embodied Knowledge: Knowing When an Organ Will Work

As I have shown, a great deal of negotiation and interpretation goes into determining what constitutes a good donor and usable parts. The clinical management of the donor body has much to do with this, yet surgeons' actual decision about whether to actually use an offered organ—the accept/ reject decision—may depend on a number of variables.

If you were using a standardized tool for a task, you would simply select any one of the several offered that met the basic parameters needed to get the job done: the right size, specifications, and so forth. You would choose the tool most readily available for offer. All you need to know is that specifications have been tested and met beforehand.

This essentially describes the way in which organs are accepted for use in the United States. As soon as donor data are reported (clinical information, medications given, laboratory data, age, cause of death, social history, medical history), surgeons make the final decision to accept or reject—usually before transplanters go to the donor hospital. Rarely did I hear reports of surgical teams rejecting an organ after arriving in the OR, except in cases in which an organ appeared to be in much worse shape upon direct inspection than diagnostic information would have predicted.

In Germany, surgeons' preliminary accept decision tends to be based on the donor's age and a few basic organ function tests. Surgeons often turn down organs over the phone, basing their decisions on the donor's age and a few organ function tests but little other donor information. One important factor, however, is where the donor is located. This concern is partly due to potential logistical difficulties: hospitals in small towns may not have heliports and be accessible only by small roads. Still, Germany is not a large country, helicopters and jets are expensive but readily available, and OR times can usually be negotiated to accommodate teams. Rather, several surgeons told me that the quality of organs can be predicted in part by the region of the country in which the donor lived. For example, they said that certain regions have more alcoholic livers or more fatty hearts.

The quality of the coordinators or the reputation of local surgeons also influences decision makers. For example, western physicians have negative perceptions about East German clinics:

"We don't like to go to [eastern region]. You can't trust that it's a good donor." (northwestern surgeon, f.n., June 1994)

"Those guys at [an eastern clinic] really don't have good technique. I've gotten kidneys from them that were really hard to transplant [due to a too-short ureter or what was perceived as badly excised vessels]." (southern surgeon, f.n., August 1994)

When an organ is shipped rather than collected personally, it is more of an unknown. This influences acceptance decisions. One surgeon told me, "I want to have the highest-quality organ. When I get it shipped to me from Eurotransplant and the organ is anonymous, then I say, 'Do we really want to [use] these?'" (f.n., October 1994). To this surgeon, what identified organs as good or bad tools was where they came from and who removed them: was it someone he knew or trusted?

I do not use these examples to generalize about all surgeons' attitudes or to suggest that practitioners treat data about organ function as unimportant. Indeed, according to one surgeon, information about the donor is the key to everything: "If you want to find out why one kidney works well and another doesn't, then you must characterize the donor. And you can't do that with three pieces of data." He was concerned because "in Germany we get very little information about the donor" (f.n., September 1994). Still, most surgeons told me that they want to see the organ and judge it for themselves within the body of the donor. For them, the decision to accept is a commitment to inspect the organ personally, not to actually take it. They make their final decision on site.

As organs are exposed during procurement, surgeons check them by sight and touch for quality—the general condition of the organ itself. Specifically, they look for the proportion of fat and structural-anatomical problems that might create trouble in the recipient. Color and texture are important to determining if the organ is damaged or diseased. Surgeons test by pressing the organ with a finger, which moves blood out of the capillaries so that they can see the tissue itself. Then they observe how quickly color returns (that is, how well the capillaries perfuse blood back into the tissue). In my observations, I noted that German surgeons spent far longer touching and looking at organs than American surgeons did (as much as five to fifteen minutes for Germans compared to less than a minute for Americans).

There are various rules of thumb for evaluating organs. For example, livers should not be "more than 50% fatty," and hearts should not be enlarged (see also Flye 1995: 58; f.n., 1994, 1995). In general, as respondents explained, livers should have a sharp edge; a rounded edge indicates swelling. Livers get harder with chronic damage—from alcohol use, in particular. Fat is determined by the number of white streaks in the organ or surrounding it and is judged independently from the overall body weight and appearance of other organs. These guidelines appear in textbooks as well as papers from scientific meetings, indicating their widespread acceptance. They are never debated, only assumed. The guidelines describe why organs change and what to look for but not how to judge the ability of the organ to function.

But how does one know if a liver is 50 percent fatty without a biopsy? How enlarged is "too enlarged"; how hard is "too hard"? When I asked German surgeons and coordinators to explain when and how an organ is rejected, they described processes based on sensory input rather than other characteristics: "Kidneys can be pretty mushy and still work." "Livers can't be too hard" (f.n., April, October 1994). In general, kidneys can be in poor condition and still work fairly well (if not, the patient can be dialyzed again), but hearts need to be in good condition.

Surgeons want to feel an organ: is it white, hard, fatty? They told me, "Even with [lab tests that measure function], it's hard to tell if an organ is really usable. Not until you see it" (f.n., September 1994). Another said, "If I just receive [an organ] in a bag, my judgment is as good as nothing. I can look at the paper and see what the [laboratory] values are, but there can be a lot wrong. The individual [visual] impression of each organ stands" (f.n., October 1994). Again, this distrust of data is sometimes tied to location. A physician coordinator in an eastern clinic claimed that many western physicians did not trust his review of the donors or the lab data: "[They say,] 'I don't care what the numbers say; I want to see it for myself'" (f.n., October 1994).

No one was able to tell me how they knew an organ, such as a liver, would work. They insisted the knowledge comes only through years of watching outcomes in transplant recipients. When I asked how they learned to discern functionality or quality, surgeons answered, "It's all emotion" or "[You learn] when you've had a thousand kidneys in your hand" (f.n., November 1995). According to Alberto Cambrosio and Peter Keating (1988), the tacit knowledge that circulates in scientific disciplines is unwritten and often impossible to articulate. This knowledge is also embedded in the practices themselves: physicians refer to personal experience, information from external sources about technique, and information about intended use during the process of scrutinizing the organ (cf. Lynch 1985, Knorr-Cetina 1981). In this sense, the surgeon's body is also a tool. His hands and eyes as sensory devices are as important as secondary representational data in diagnosing the condition of the organ and predicting whether it will function for the intended use.

Palpating and scrutinizing an organ individualizes it and places decision making squarely at this point rather than earlier in the process. Relying on this type of knowledge rather than standardized measures of function makes German practice seem more craftlike than American practice. Organs may have theoretical threshold limits of function: "A normal kidney has maybe 1 million nephrons. If 100,000 don't work, the kidney can still function. This is its reserve capacity" (f.n., July 1994). Yet respondents often spoke of functionality as an inherent part of each individual and unique organ. As one coordinator told me, "each organ has its own reserve capacity" (f.n., July 1994).

In addition to considering individual characteristics, surgeons also judge an organ based on its intended purpose. I often heard them evaluate an organ's functionality by estimating how it would function in a particular recipient. These different ways of evaluating can happen simultaneously, as my field notes show:

> The liver surgeon is holding up the liver before dissecting it. He presses his finger against the surface. It is swollen. The other surgeon thinks it's okay, but the first surgeon continues to grope underneath. He finds a tear.

They discuss the recipient. They discuss whether the liver could either be sectioned or repaired. The liver might not begin functioning right away. Also, the recipient is in poor physical shape and an older man. If the liver began to bleed in the recipient, he might not recover. After about fifteen minutes, they decide not to take the liver after all. (f.n., October 1994)

When discussing organs and judging their quality, surgeons often refer to the regenerative capability of the tissue. If the tissue is from a younger donor, for example, it can recover and regenerate in the recipient even if badly damaged. From my field notes:

The liver is very bruised, and the color is a bit off [from trauma]. The surgeon checks for bleeding. Everything seems okay except for swelling. He runs his hand under the liver, presses on top. He gently pulls it upward. He stops and looks, moving his face closer to the surface. The surgeon talks constantly with other members of liver team. He pauses a moment, asks for a double perfusion setup. Then he runs his hands along the surface and the edge again. He stands up and pulls back. He discusses with other surgeons if the liver is too bruised and swollen. Then he begins to dissect arteries. He checks underneath with his hand again. More discussion. More dissection in situ. The recipient is an adult, very ill, but not high-urgency status. The surgeon decides that since the donor is a child, the liver will probably regenerate well. (f.n., October 1994)

Materials are thus matched to the intended purpose based on perceptions of quality and usability. Yet unlike the United States, decision making in Germany is not based on characteristics of the donor's person as described by his social history (except in cases of known severe alcoholism, when the organ is rejected at the offer stage). Medical history and test data also figure less prominently than they do in the United States. Surgeons do not usually ask for laboratory data during the evaluation process, nor do they inquire about the donor's smoking, drinking, or health habits. Instead, they combine types of knowledge to make their judgments: representational data, tactual and visual observations, and knowledge of the intended recipient. In short, even though the organ is individualized, it is not personalized: a heart is not a part removed from a juvenile delinquent or a kind and generous housewife.

If the organ is intended for research, quality is not so critical. In fact, most research material comes from organs rejected for transplantation. In livers, for example, individual cells are more important than the whole organ because the tissue may be broken down to the cellular level in any case. Researchers are likely to reject livers with poor enzyme data or those that might be physically damaged because of trauma or too-long warm ischemic time.

Interestingly, I visited three clinics where new technology was being tested that purportedly could evaluate the function and characteristics of organs. Rather than test organ function as screening tests did in earlier stages of evaluating the donor, several of these devices were applied directly to the organ after it was exposed in the OR. For example, one model had a membrane surface that, when it touched the tissue, registered certain enzymes and chemical levels. Another device tested liver function before surgery, fiberoptically measuring how well the liver could clear a dye. The coordinator hoped this device could prevent the problem of having teams show up to inspect the liver and then reject it based on physical appearance. He was planning a trial in which the device's measurements would be correlated with a surgeon's visual inspection. He had no access, however, to precise outcome data (which transplant clinics do not widely disseminate), so he could not correlate diffusion rates with outcomes (however one defines them).

This is a fascinating scenario. The DSO paid for the device's evaluation. The company marketing it wants to promote the device based on the promise that it will cost less than sending a helicopter with a team to look at an organ likely to be rejected. (The cost is 60,000 marks, plus 300 marks for a disposable catheter.)[6] The device could also be used for living patients—telling if, and in which category, a liver patient should be listed for transplantation. Although not every hospital can afford to buy the equipment, the DSO argues that enough could be bought to share within regions; and the DSO-employed coordinator could bring the device to any hospital, even those with minimal diagnostic equipment of their own. Of course, this would require a centralized organization to pay for the equipment and regional suborganizations to provide such diagnostic services to hospitals. By enabling regional coordinators to monitor patients with this and other equipment at the bedside, the DSO could solidify its control.

Thus, local practices of decision making (the need to see and touch tissue) have consequences for other actors (waste of time and tissue) and offer an opportunity for new actors to enter the arena and profit. At the same time, employing this technology and its necessary infrastructure enhances the purposes of a central managing body, increases control, and solidifies the power base. The technology is meant to standardize practice and provide quantifiable measures of quality that may in turn affect local practices of decision making. Through these subtle organizational and economic changes, power shifts in ways that are rarely visible to the public.

Removing and Processing the Materials

Organs are clamped off and then flushed with special cold solutions to cool and begin preserving the tissue. But organ excision becomes tricky when major shared vessels and other structures must be separated to be removed. This can create conflict among surgical teams about how to proceed. For example, heart surgeons want to clamp in a way that prevents the liver preservation solution from getting into the heart because it contains potassium, which will affect heart function. Abdominal teams prefer to flush through the inferior vena cava to prevent fluid from obscuring the abdominal visual field. This, however, can flood the pericardium and obscure the thoracic visual field. Likewise, liver and pancreas teams should agree on the level of division of celiac and superior mesenteric artery branches because these organs share the celiac axis. Vessels, like ureters from the kidney, must not be cut too short, or there will not be enough left to reattach in the recipient.

The heart is removed first, then lungs (if taken), and then abdominal organs, with kidneys last. This is the order in which tissue is most to least damaged by lack of oxygen after the aorta is clamped to remove the heart. Heart removal is the most dramatic moment of the procedure. After initial preparation and clamping of vessels, cardioplegic solution is injected to stop the action of the heart muscle. The tempo of work increases as the time nears for final clamping of the major arteries. Abdominal team members usually pause and stand back until the final clamping is done. The anesthesiologist becomes more active, often moving around to check progress while carefully monitoring hemodynamic responses. The exact time of clamping is announced loudly and marked by the circulator and the coordinator on procedure forms. Known as cross-clamp time, this moment is important because it marks the beginning of ischemic time—the interval when there is no blood circulating oxygen to all organs and tissues.[7] The heart team moves quickly to finish removal and leaves in a rather dramatic rush.

As they are being freed from their bodily moorings of ligaments and vessels, organs are cooled with iced saline slush, usually dumped into thoracic and abdominal cavities in large quantities. Toward the end of the procedure, the spleen is removed and cut into sections for the receiving transplant centers and for a central tissue typing lab (if available). Lymph nodes may also be removed for testing. Artificial life support measures are then discontinued, and the constant beeping of monitors ceases. The room becomes quieter; the pace remains steady but less intense.

After removal, organs are again checked physically for abnormalities. Kidneys are perfused with preservation fluid to check flow and function, which is then rated and recorded on the procurement form. This work is often performed by surgeons and coordinators together: one person must operate the bag with perfusion fluid, while the other checks the appearance of the kidney. Occasionally I was included in this process: "The surgeon turns to me and asks me to run perfusion lines for the kidneys. At first I reach for the wrong line. It should be obvious which is which, but I was flustered by the request. I get it going slowly, and it runs okay. The kidneys appear to perfuse well, and after about two minutes the surgeon gives them a high rating" (f.n., November 1995).

Additional dissection and preparation may be performed after removal, although German surgeons often do this in the body. Newer and now more standard techniques include an en bloc removal of kidneys as well as the liver. Some European coordinators and surgeons complain about German techniques, saying they take too long and are old-fashioned: "A coordinator from another country whispers to me, 'These Germans are so *slow*— they're famous for taking so long. Everyone else uses [a standardized technique]. In five years you will never see this anymore. Livers will be removed en bloc and dissected at the back table. Only the Germans still do this nonsense'" (f.n., October 1994).

Overhearing this comment, the coordinator from the German team came over to me and explained that taking the extra time and doing more precision work made for a much better-functioning organ and a better outcome for the recipient. This is another example of the Germans' craftlike approach: a raw material is sculpted and prepared for use rather than treated as a mass-produced item or part not meant to have interim processing. From my field notes:

> The coordinator is at the back table, meticulously trimming extra fat and tissue away from the kidney and arranging the ureters. He works slowly and seems slightly annoyed that I am watching and taking notes. It is like someone doing fine woodcarving: he visualizes first, then works in one area—carefully slicing a small section away, then a bit more. He seems to be concerned with how it looks. He moves ureters gently back and forth and measures them. This takes at least fifteen minutes. I have never seen this much detail work in the United States. The kidneys are on top of a cold surface but not submerged in iced saline, so I wonder about how [the team is] counting warm ischemic time. (f.n., July 1994)

Because the kidneys were not on ice for a longer period of time, this style of working might have sacrificed tissue quality for preparation and work quality.

After preparation, each organ is placed in iced saline in a plastic bag, surrounded by two more bags filled with iced saline, and then packed in an ice chest for transport. The procedure up to this point usually takes one and a half to two hours—less if only one organ is removed, more if there are complications or if a team is slow to arrive.

Organs rejected for transplant, the leftover spleen, and other parts removed but not used are supposed to be put back inside the body cavity before closing, although at this point tissue is sometimes kept out for research. The body is often closed with cheaper or less aesthetic material than is used for living patients. It is becoming common in the United States to use surgical staples, which are faster than suturing and will not be seen. Closure is often left to junior members of the team—on occasion, to someone from the host hospital. It is considered extremely impolite in the United States to leave this duty to the house staff. The coordinator often oversees body closure or helps to close it herself. The body is then cleaned of excess disinfectant and blood. As a courtesy, the coordinator and the assistants from American explanting teams help the host hospital staff clean up the OR. In Germany, however, this job is done almost entirely by the housekeeping staff.

In both the United States and Germany, I offered to help with final body preparations and room cleanup. American coordinators were surprised but accepted gladly. Afterward, I was treated much more as an insider and with more respect. (I overheard one coordinator telling another one about my offer, portraying it very positively.) In Germany, I was told firmly that cleanup was the job of housekeeping and staff nurses and that I should not help—another example of the country's rigid medical hierarchy.

The body is frequently left alone in the room after the teams are done, something that would never occur with a live patient. Occasionally, workers from the host hospital will enter and begin cleaning the room during the last phases of closure. As tubes (intubation, IV, catheters) are removed and the body is uncovered, the donor again emerges as a human body rather than an object being worked on. Now, however, the usual signs of death are clearer. Air may rush out of the lungs and collected moisture evacuate from the nose and mouth. Within a few minutes after the aorta is clamped, cessation of blood flow becomes visible: a yellowish, waxy appearance replaces pinker flesh tones, and purplish blotches show where blood pools on the underside of the body. Two German coordinators described their perceptions of this point:

"This is the worst moment. The patient lies there, and everyone is gone. This is a cold, lonely way to die." (southern coordinator, f.n., November 1994)

"Now he is dead for me. He looks, feels, and smells like a dead person. He is once again whole." (eastern coordinator, f.n., December 1993)

These words speak volumes about the double meanings of the body at death for all participants, even among coordinators whose work is deeply committed to transplantation. For American coordinators, who had been so involved with the donors and their identities, this point was a natural conclusion to the course of events and provided closure. After working closely with the physical body in various states of being covered or connected to technologies, digitized into data, and otherwise converted into a preserver-container for the organs, they saw the body as being returned to its appropriate state. For the German coordinators, however, this was often the point of rupture and, except for the occasional times when they dealt with the donor's family, was often the time that they were most able to see the body as a person. Surgeons have a different relationship to the body than do co-ordinators in either the United States or Germany since their focus is on the recipient and they approach the donor only briefly and then primarily as a source of therapeutic tools. For them it may be more possible to say, as Foucault (1975) did, that the surface of the body disappears and that the organs are seen in isolation according to the model put forth by the atlas—knowledge produced by the cadaver. For coordinators and other partici-pants, the relations among the body as subject, object, and tool are more complex.

If tissue is to be removed in the OR, tissue procurement teams wait at least until closing begins. This new group of actors can be technicians, pa-thologists, specialists (such as ophthalmologists or orthopedists), or oth-ers associated with tissue banking. Corneas are most easily removed if the entire eyeball is taken out and brought elsewhere, but they can also be re-moved while the eyes are in the body. Plastic caps are inserted either here or at the morgue to replace the eye shape. Skin is removed in long sec-tions—from the lower back, upper thigh, or inner arm. Bones are removed from the lower arm or upper leg. This can be a difficult procedure for ev-eryone involved, especially since the body is now more visible: more clearly dead, yet more obviously a human being. From my notes:

[A physician on trauma call arrives in the last half-hour of the procedure to take corneas.] This guy is young. He seems afraid of what he's doing, taking tentative plucks and jabs at the eye ligaments, then stopping and looking away frequently. His face is very red. . . . He replaces the eyeball with a gauze wad before doing the next eye [rather than finishing and then replacing both at the same time]. Each eye goes into a small plastic container filled with fluid. . . . He labels everything carefully and then leaves quickly. While he works, another surgeon is looking for the spleen. The donor has already been extubated and lines removed. Drapes are also partly off, so we can see most of the body. Blood is pooling underneath. OR nurses have gone or are working in a subroom. (f.n., October 1995)

Many tissues can be removed up to two days after death and are handled by pathologists in the hospital morgue, where autopsies are performed. As I discussed in chapter 6, they are rarely procured in the OR. Tissue pro-curement adds considerable time to the overall procedure. For some people, it can be difficult to observe because of the necessary degree of invasion.

In particular, it involves considerable defacing of recognizable human features, such as skin, eyes, and ears. For these reasons, and because tissue procurement requires further planning and organization with more teams, coordinators do not always make the extra effort to contact tissue banks or try to arrange for tissues to be removed in the morgue after organ procurement—even when permission to procure tissues has been granted.

After all OR procedures are finished, the body is cleaned and prepared for the morgue. In the United States, the hands are tied, the jaw strapped shut, and any remaining tubes removed. Absorbent pads are placed under the buttocks and sometimes over the incision and mouth to absorb leaking fluids. The house staff or the coordinator usually covers the body with a plastic shroud. In Germany, the body is not prepared at all in the OR; it is covered loosely with a sheet and sent to the morgue, where other workers do the cadaver handling.

After the body leaves the OR, the pace of work slows:

Now comes a let-down time as activities begin to slow and the tension and pace decrease. There is often more informal talking and some rehashing of the case, especially if coordinators from more than one center are present. It occurred to me that this is the only place and time when coordinators have much contact with each other, aside from the single annual meeting for those who participate in the DSO. Like dressing before the procedure, a different social space is created to decompress after an intense experience requiring considerable concentration and management of the presentation of self. Afterward everyone moves to the changing room. (Again, there is only one room.) Some shower and ask if I want to as well. There is only a curtain partition to the room where others are undressing, so I am sure I can hear some of the aftertalk if I do shower; and after all, it's 2:30 A.M. and I've been on this case since 7:30 yesterday morning. (f.n., July 1994)

The work is not over for the coordinator, who must phone data to transplant centers, follow up on any other test results, advise UNOS or ET of the outcome, finish the paperwork, and prepare and arrange for shipping organs not taken with the teams. (Sometimes teams will remove organs that will be sent to transplant centers that have not sent their own teams.) This adds another hour and a half to his work.

It is common for American coordinators to phone another person from the OPO, either as a debriefing buddy or, just as important, to keep them awake on the long drive home after an intense situation that may have lasted for more than twenty-four hours (Hogle 1996). There is no such system in Germany, although the coordinators I observed occasionally called a coworker from their transplant center or talked extensively—and far more personally than usual—with me afterward. This is when I often heard stories of other cases or similar difficult situations and listened to ruminations and criticism of surgeons' techniques.

Unlike American coordinators, Germans did not discuss the donor or the recipient, but sometimes they did discuss the appearance or condition of the organ. If an organ was rejected, they often replayed the decision, mulling over whether the tissue was viable or if it could have worked in the recipient.

Culture and Medical Practices

As these examples show, scientific knowledge is adapted to local conditions and ways of using knowledge, and nonroutine situations create new sets of contingencies that must be managed. Practices vary and produce different outcomes within particular systems of culture and power. As David Hess (1995: 53) says, "actors come to networks within cultures that provide them with biases about appropriate forms of knowledge, methodology and machinery." The point I want to stress here is that, while structures and institutions play a clear role in the social relations of HBM technologies, the sheer materiality of the body is also involved in producing knowledge and practices.

The U.S. practice of using techniques to convert information about quality and functionality into quantifiable representational data suggests that the expertise lies in the ability to collect, interpret, and manage information produced by visual and sensory machine technologies. Also, the extensive clinical and narrative data collected about the donor create an object that is known beforehand. Relying upon such information means that practitioners can decide to reject or accept an organ in relatively standard and routine ways—and at some distance from the donor. This also makes it possible to share the information among many "experts" who are both communicators of information and producers of knowledge. If the data are interpretable according to predetermined standards and definitions of normal function, then they may not require a surgeon (or even a medically trained person, for that matter) alone either to transmit information or to make the decision.[8]

Focusing on this type of data and at this stage is consistent with the idea of being able to adjust the tool through the kinds of constant interventions in the donor management and preservation process as discussed in chapter 8. Employing technologies to change the characteristics of individual and varying tissue creates a more standardized, technological object. Thus, it is not as critical to use a variety of decision-making skills because the organ can be predicted to function similarly in different recipients. Even when it doesn't, further interventions can be applied later in the body of the recipient. The interchangeability of participants and materials is consistent with a system that functions over a very large geographical area, has a greater volume of procedures than do other countries, and has a stable infrastructure that includes rapid transportation and communication technologies.

German practices of relying on direct experience and sensory processes as well as more attention to detailed finish work produce a therapeutic tool that is different from those created in the American process. German culture favors the precise, the orderly, the meticulous.[9] Germans are well known for their highly skilled precision work. Industries in which these characteristics are important (automobiles, machine tools, scientific instruments, optics) flourished in Germany in the nineteenth and twentieth centuries. Workers in many fields are trained extensively in the minutiae of techniques: apprentice machinists may practice a single polishing technique for a month, a housekeeper may have four years of training to work in a hotel, medical students are required to have far more hands-on experience with certain techniques than they would be in other countries. Thus, slow, careful, methodical precision, with attention to manual skills, both in judging organs for use and in dissecting and preparing them, is consistent with other ways of working in German society.[10]

Such practices also reconfirm the image of German medicine that respondents expressed to me: highly skilled, well trained, competent. Medical education in Germany and the structure of medical practice in hospitals are institutional influences on the way knowledge is drawn upon as well as who is seen to be a credible source of knowledge. The same technologies and data sources are available to German physicians and surgeons, but training often favors additional sources of knowledge, much of which is passed on from mentoring professor to student.

In organ procurement, knowledge about the donor as a source comes from basic clinical data but also from knowing the physicians at that hospital, who might be identified with it in terms of quality of care, and knowing where (which region) the donor came from. But the primary focus is on knowledge produced from the interiors of the body—knowledge held by fewer participants, who are given the authority to make a judgment about the quality of a body's parts. There are far fewer experts who could know and learn the skill necessary to sense when a liver is too fatty, a kidney too mushy. Even the coordinators, for whom this work is a livelihood, do not have this authority, nor are they given credibility as a source of knowledge. Instead, they are the invisible workers who make the arrangements and follow the protocols to make the procurement happen.[11]

German medical professionals were quick to point out that many American transplant practices are far too reckless and unethical. They base that judgment largely on what they perceive as too commercial an orientation. A number of American surgeons champion aggressive, industrial techniques for managing procurement, which many Germans consider to be inappropriate for medical practice. One such technique was the creation of technologies to preserve or change the characteristics of organs in situ. Respondents called this idea "absurd" or "a waste of money." A craftlike, less industrial approach projects an image of authentic and traditional medical delivery, with more care given to the work itself.

In contrast to U.S. efforts to create highly processed, standard tissue products, human materials are treated in Germany like natural objects naturally produced. By conserving the natural, individual, and inherent characteristics of each organ, German physicians believe that they better maintain the functionality, quality, use value, and perceived viability for the intended recipient. Using manual and sensory skills to detect these qualities reinforces this idea of natural technique. By not using more standardized, industrialized techniques, surgeons distance themselves from administrative means and objectified data, handle organs more as individual and unique entities, and perhaps in doing so project an image of practicing medicine with pietätsempfinden rather than procuring tools. At the same time, they retain and restrict expertise.

The explanations I have offered here are only part of the picture; there are many other contextual variables. In the United States, for example, the push to increase the number of liver procedures due to certification requirements means an orientation toward quantity rather than outcomes (Hogle 1992).[12] To get the numbers up, workers must procure more livers, including less optimal ones (f.n., February 1992). That is, more livers from marginal (older, sicker) donors are used, as are livers in poorer condition, than would be if the work were oriented strictly toward outcomes. Because of the treatments and technologies available for recipients (which insurers cover frequently and often fully), problems that arise can be fixed later. In Germany, payment has not been a limitation, so this pressure does not exist.[13] Thus, in the United States, much of the push comes from attempts to increase the number of procedures to build expertise and further standardize and perfect techniques that are thought to produce better (more reproducible and therefore more fundable) results. The response to the shortage of organs is more aggressive pursuit of donors (Hogle 1995b).

German practice is oriented toward outcomes in the recipient, although the reasons are different from those in the United States. The most obvious difference is the division of labor. U.S. procurement coordinators are distinct from transplant coordinators who work with potential recipients. They are employed in free-standing, not-for-profit organizations separated from transplant interests. In Germany, coordinators are physically located in transplant clinics and deal with both donors and recipients. As I have mentioned, coordinators keep photos of potential recipients in their offices, and patients on the waiting list occasionally visit them in their offices.

The majority of U.S. coordinators are intensive care nurses accustomed to hands-on care of patients, whereas most coordinators in Germany are physicians. This alone, however, is insufficient to explain differences in practice: German coordinators who were not physicians also did not participate in hands-on care of brain-dead patients to the same extent that U.S. coordinators do.

In a setting of high controversy—within the ranks and in the public domain—it becomes especially important to prove the value and efficacy of contentious technologies. Germany's graft survival rates are quite high (Eurotransplant 1993, 1994; Deutsches Stiftung für Organspende 1993). Combining close, direct inspection with meticulous preparation and dissecting techniques may be slow and less standard, but it allows surgeons to craft and tailor a therapeutic device for a specific user. The extensive handling and inspection of the organ may also lead surgeons to be more conservative or cautious in their choice, which may in turn affect the outcome. It is counterintuitive to reject marginal organs in a time of severe shortage, and I do not suggest that German surgeons reject organs without good reason. Rather, since it is not possible to pursue donors more aggressively, each donor must be used carefully. An enlightening study would be to compare rejection and waste rates with offers and then to compare that finding to rates in other countries.

Still, there are unanswered questions about the perceptions and politics of outcomes. Graft and patient survival depends on a wide variety of variables, including the condition of the transplanted patient, her aftercare, and the surgeon's technique in addition to the quality of the transplanted organ.[14] Moreover, tissue changes during preservation in the phase between removal from the donor and implantation.[15] Can extensive sensory input and focus on organs in situ really predict an organ's ability to function in the new body? Will they predict the effect of tissue changes on the health and survival of the recipient? There is clearly cultural filtering in the use, choice, and interpretation of data meant to predict future outcomes. To what extent, if any, will these practices change with pressures to align with European (and globalized) techniques and knowledge bases?

German practices may have interesting implications for organizational and scientific theories. As I have mentioned, the length of donor holding time before procurement is quite short in Germany. By refusing to use techniques that could extend this time period, practitioners uphold the need to keep organs within nearby regions. They maintain the popular conception of urgency since without preservation techniques both the body and the organs will fail. But with less time to find an optimal recipient, they must choose a good-enough local one. This supports justifications to develop and maintain regional networks and keep organs locally. I see the practice as another form of resistance to the HLA system, which requires an institutionalized organization at the national or international level to establish a large pool of optimal matches. Thus, the argument to donate organs in Germany—to help local and particular others—is supported. In fact, a few transplant centers publish newsletters or news releases that advertise the number of organs kept and transplanted into local patients compared to those sent to other regions. One coordinator in a center that does follow HLA guidelines argued, "[HLA matching] means that too many organs go outside our area. This makes it hard to convince families to donate" (f.n., May 1994).

By observing actual activities, one can witness the contingent nature of technical work. The adaptation of tools and techniques and the use of various bases of knowledge demonstrate how components interact to shape local practices. While they exist within a specific technical domain, these practices clearly are constituted within broader social, organizational, technoscientific, and economic contexts.

Ten

Conclusions

Medicine and the Politics of Redemption

During my last few days in Germany, I went on a long hike in the Harz mountains, which lie at the heart of German legends and ancient history. Stimulated by both the beauty of the landscape and conversations with friends, I did not mark how far we had gone, or how far we still had to go, until my body began to tell me that I had not been fully prepared for the distance. It was nightfall when we emerged from the path and groped toward the light of the open lodge door. My tiredness felt good—the strain of assimilating images, the ache of feeling more connected to the things and people I would soon have to leave.

Back in Berlin two days later, I felt excruciating pain in my knees, and within hours I was unable to walk. I left Germany in a wheelchair, a symbol of differentness that marked me as an outsider. My problem was later diagnosed as osteomalacia, a softening of the bone and cartilage in which the tissue shatters into a million tiny fragments upon physical shock. It is the process of reabsorbing and metabolizing the minuscule particles and reforming new tissue from osteoids that causes the pain.

The parallel to my fieldwork experience is not subtle. I had no idea at the outset how far and through what sort of terrain I would have to go—partly hostile, partly wonderful. I left the experience feeling in some ways even more unclear about what I was seeing than I had when I began.

Germany, too, has had its shocks. The fragile and late-born idea of building identity on the concept of nation was shattered by World War II so that it is no longer possible to speak of Germany without evoking stark images of power and inhumanity. As one respondent wondered, "just how many decades are necessary before the world forgets the sins of my grandfather and begins to see me as a person who lives and works in Germany, and not as a perpetrator?" (f.n., December 1994). Today, the terms *community* and *greater good of society* are rarely used in public discourse. Just who constitutes the moral community in Germany today? How many immigrants can the country absorb without destroying the infrastructure that Germans have worked so hard to rebuild after the war? Are some residents more authentically German than others? Should they be privileged over or have more rights than others? These questions overlap problems arising from reunification. The "separate but equal" mentality of early unification has given way to mutual distaste, blame, and anger between East and West Germans.

With the backdrop of scientific and social projects designed to purify the body of *das Volk,* should Germans be allowed to compete with other industrialized nations in biotechnology and genetics research? Are the policing of the Gene Law and restrictions on certain medical practices a necessary price to pay for past wrongs, and can such checks create either an institutional or cultural change in the social relations of knowledge production?[1] These issues divide Germans into generations, regions, ideologies, and political factions. They are questions addressed not only by Germans but by the world.

Thus, on the one hand, Germany resists reformulating previous support structures; on the other, it struggles with pressing political, economic, and social needs to unify direction and action. And just when the federal government tries to glue these disparate bits together, a new trauma fragments social material in a new way. Reforms of symbolically loaded social policy (health care, immigration laws, abortion rights, social welfare), a new German presence in European and world politics, scandals about the treatment of individuals, the resurgence of neo-Nazi and Communist movements: each jarring revelation seems to atomize the structure of postwar and postunification society. Germany is incorporating the new while metabolizing the old: the pain is in the reabsorption.

Sharing, Giving, and Entitlement to Public Goods

In his work on the relation of self to society, Louis Dumont (1986) describes the distinct form that Germany took in comparison with other European countries. According to Dumont, the state in Germany has historically been conceptualized not as a protector of individuals' rights and liberties (as in France) but as an embodiment of the whole of society: an expression of the collective individual rather than a collective of individuals. Germans see themselves as being German first, and any rights or liberties must be subordinated to what is necessary to belong to that society. Dumont compares this notion to the French history of legal concepts of individual human dignity and worth, which suggests that rights are inherent by virtue of being human regardless of nation or collectivity. Here he notes, however, the influence of Luther, who recognized the necessity of the political community while subordinating matters of the state to matters of the individual spirit. This has left an important legacy in religious and social life in Germany, particularly in considering the issue of dignity and the individual's ability to assert herself against the social or political order.

Until its first unification in 1871, Germany existed not as whole society but as a collection of states and principalities that did not even have a common language until the end of the sixteenth century. This had a lasting legacy: economic policy, health, welfare, and other protections have been governed at local and regional levels rather than federally. Not until the rise of National Socialism did Germans have a strong sense of being an integrated social body. After World War II and the partition of states, it became anathema to speak of social body or national identity except as a nostalgic hope of reunifying east and west. As Diana Forsythe (1989) notes, the period of greatest German nationalism and social unity was a time that most Germans today wish had never taken place.

The Basic Law of 1949 affirmed the dignity and worth of persons and thus provided an official document of remediation for past wrongs. The law and its related penal codes and institutions that followed laid out what constitutes a violation to persons and bodies. But what constitutes violence to—and inviolability of—persons and their bodies for political and legal purposes may differ from what is seen as necessary or desirable for scientists wanting to maintain standing in their own institutions as well as international communities, economic stakeholders competing in global markets, and individuals considering the fate of their bodies as they encounter the medical-industrial complex. Concerns about the right of medical and state authorities to intervene in private bodies in modernity, along with old questions about the nature of the dead body and its relation to personal identity, come into play.

The body in late twentieth-century Germany is laden with multiple meanings; it is both a biological being and a culturally produced entity. Debates about individuals' obligation to donate organs and tissues for the good of society and the right of the state to claim these materials have made the brain-dead body a political symbol as well. Proposals to allow the procurement of human materials without consent have dramatized concerns about the encroachment of medicine and the state on the interests—and bodies—of individuals.

Since the Basic Law was written, technological innovations intended to extend lives have complicated matters. The private process of dying has come under the stewardship of public institutions and legislatures. The authors of the Basic Law considered the rights and duties toward the dead before this era of rapidly increasing health care costs and large numbers of the aged and chronically ill who survive. The pressures of economic forces; the technological imperative to extend certain lives; the interest in competitive, lucrative industries and research opportunities have involved a reconceptualization of persons, bodies, and rights. In this change, many people in Germany see the wolf waiting by the herd of sheep.

Jean Baudrillard (1993) has said that in earlier ages death was visible but uncontrollable. Today, we can stage, extend, and manipulate the timing and manner of death; death is no longer "normal." Baudrillard asserts that because death is now subject to science and technology, a new sort of social contract arises that makes it possible to say that society as a whole is collectively responsible for the death of individuals. It follows, then, that meanings of individuals' deaths—both biological and social—are ascribed. Previously, there was a different sense of identity and social life; in an era when there was no concept of social good, bodies were not given or donated to any purpose altruistically. Now life and everything in it has to be given a meaning—what Zygmunt Bauman (1992) calls a distribution of freedoms and dependencies that gives meaning to survival. Through organ donation, medicine takes on the role of deciding how distribution and sharing should proceed in a society. Formalized institutions and practices become sites for negotiations over how to allocate scarce organs and tissues and who is entitled to human materials as a public resource.[2] At the same time, survival in the context of giving and using one's body after death constitutes a particular type of immortality—that is, the memory of a reimagined life and its continued animation in another body and the ongoing life or survival of another person.

The death that Baudrillard describes is a secularized one. Yet transplant communities, most notably those in the United States, have been quite successful in reframing the use of parts from the dead in quasi-religious terms. Slogans such as "give the gift of life" and promotional images of living again evoke themes of resurrection that tie notions of continued animation of donated materials to the born-again life of the recipient (Hogle 1992). The act of resurrecting is linked to the act of sacrifice; individuals are encouraged to share bodily parts they will no longer need after death.

But converting bodily remains—organic waste—to something medically useful creates multiple types of redemption. As I showed in chapter 2, the act of donation can allow a life perceived by some to be useless to serve a social good. I often heard this rationale in the United States, particularly when the donor had been involved in criminal or even questionable activities. For example, several coordinators told me they most often got permission to take the organs of children when the death was caused by child abuse.

Ironically, this "useless life" defense was used by doctors in the Nuremberg trials at the end of World War II. Rationalizing their treatment of camp prisoners, defendants suggested that "by being injected, frozen or transplanted, subjects could cleanse themselves of their crimes" (Caplan 1992: 266). The same arguments are used to justify the execution of Chinese prison inmates and using their kidneys for transplants.

While observing organ procurement in the United States, I noted that families' reasons for donating organs related to "helping with grieving" or "making something meaningful out of the death." Attempting to persuade family members to donate a loved one's organs, procurement coordinators frequently argued that donation was a good way to memorialize the dead (Hogle 1992, 1996). In the rituals and rhetoric created around American organ donation, the act of donating becomes an act of commemoration. Special celebrations and memorial services are sponsored by organ procurement organizations in honor of donors and their families, sporting events display the vigor of organ recipients, and narratives circulate about altruism and good will.[3] Providing tissue to others thus becomes a way of depositing memories and ensuring continuation and immortality.

The message of organ donation as an ongoing gift of life has been adopted by the international transplant community. The theme conveys the idea that while the donor cannot survive in his existing form, he can live through the biological survival of another person. The conversion of one person's body parts to life-saving therapy in the body of another is represented discursively as a natural flow—the process of cycling from death to life. At the same time, the gift becomes a legacy of the donor as an identity—an altruistic, generous person who would want others to survive.

While most of this universal rhetoric has also been used in Germany, meanings have been received and interpreted quite differently. In German promotional campaigns (of which there are few), the message is inverted: those who fail to donate are selfish and wasteful. Organs are seen as material goods that should be passed on to others when not in use. Promotion focuses less on ongoing life, especially for specific individuals, and more on contributing to society. One advertisement featured a body being buried with money and luxury items such as stereo equipment and an expensive car. The narrative suggested that taking such goods—including organs that could be used by others—was wasteful. When this ad was previewed at the annual meeting of the DSO, it invoked a variety of reactions. While some transplant coordinators applauded the message, many felt that it was distasteful and inappropriate and would damage efforts to portray organ donation as a charitable activity. Ironically, the theme of greed, often applied to medical professionals, was in this case thrown back on the public.

German discourse about organ and tissue donation often contains two terms: *Solidarität* (solidarity) in the east and *Nächstenliebe* (Christian charity) in the west. Solidarität has specific connotations related to Socialist ideas of working together toward common goals. Respondents told me that members of society have a duty to share body parts: "We should share the profits in a society" (f.n., December 1993). Nächstenliebe, on the other hand, has specifically religious connotations of giving and sharing. More voluntary than solidarity, it still indicates a responsibility (rather than a duty) to others. Members of society are encouraged to donate organs to needy people to fulfill a social and personal religious need for contributing something to others. West German donor families describe a feeling of wanting to share. While they do not direct this desire toward particular individuals, they often want body parts to go someone in their own region.

What exactly do notions of solidarity, charity, individualism, and selfishness mean in Germany today? I had a sense from many eastern respondents that individualism—equated with egotism—is a capitalist characteristic contaminating the east. West Germans blame bad influences from the United States and a decline in traditional German moral standards for what they perceive as a new trend toward selfishness and aggression. Among Germans from all regions, there is a tension between the nostalgia of sharing to create greater social cohesion and competition for their own fair share. With large numbers of immigrants and the addition of new German states, there is growing disgruntlement about sharing jobs, public money and services, child care spaces, housing, and other goods.

Thus, attempts to convince the German public and medical professionals that donating organs contributes to the social good are fraught with problems. To use bodily materials without depicting procurement practices as violations necessitates a careful balance of needs and benefits, with some appearance of having everything under control.

Interdisciplinary Studies of Science, Technology, and Medicine

At the beginning of this chapter, I described my journey through harrowing yet wondrous territory, with unexpected results. And so it goes for the researcher trying to traverse academic disciplines. In recent years, there has been increasing interest in combining perspectives from anthropology and the social study of science, technology, and medicine.[4] Anthropology has long observed health and illness, healers and therapies but has only lately expanded its purview to include laboratory science and the making of medical technologies. Science and technology studies have for some three decades focused on the interior workings and exterior politics of science, including medicine. Since the mid-1980s, they have increasingly turned to ethnographic techniques for studying scientific communities. Joining these perspectives has helped us understand that culture permeates science just as science permeates everyday life.

Using an interdisciplinary structure reframes the study of health and illness, showing how "normal," "pathological," and "dying" are given new meanings through particular technologies and how these meanings are used (or unused or adapted) by various participants. Rayna Rapp's (1988) work on amniocentesis is exemplary in this regard, demonstrating how technology is read in contexts of race and class. Margaret Lock (1995), too, demonstrates fundamental differences in what it means to be human in various cultural contexts along with ways in which public and professional discourses of brain death are constructed.

These examples, among others, have made an important contribution by showing how knowledge is a social product. George Marcus and Michael Fischer (1986) and others who critique and reformulate ethnographic research have pointed out that such knowledge is produced in many sites. New knowledge is incorporated into peoples' lives in material ways: consider a woman who prophylactically removes her breasts if she tests positive for a gene; a man who must sort out whether to get a myoelectric arm or a simple prosthesis to replace his lost limb—which can he afford and what work will he be able to do? A person who is told that depression or hyperactivity is biologically based must decide whether to medicate the problem or examine alternative explanations or solutions—and deal with the implications of a changed personality.

But by focusing on either the patient's world or the technology alone, researchers often miss important connections: the fact that this is not necessarily an autonomous subject according to the way we define this in the United States; the question of how the technology will be paid for; what and whose interests are at stake in selecting a particular technology over alternatives; what kinds of tools, techniques, and people are involved in its development and use. The ways these processes involve selecting and applying certain knowledge bases need further study. Emily Martin (1998: 28) points to the limitations of exclusionary science and technology studies, asking, "What if network building and resource accumulation are not the only way knowledge is established? What if many other kinds of processes proceeding from fundamentally different assumptions about the world profoundly affect experts and scientists even as they accumulate resources and build networks?"

I have said little directly about bioethics, my other concern in studying complex medical technologies. Philosophical, legal, and policy analyses have all exhaustively considered organ donation and transplantation; brain death and the implicated issues of death and dying; justice in access and allocation; and other related inquiries. I hope that contributions from social scientists, particularly those with ethnographic detail, will continue to flesh out these structural frames. In particular, I hope that work will move beyond Euro-American representations of all individuals as autonomous free agents and look harder at the less visible patterns and infrastructures that affect choice, including much-needed perspectives on race, class, gender, and position in relation to industrialized western societies.[5]

I see further tantalizing possibilities for explaining knowledge production in interdisciplinary legal studies. Sheila Jasanoff (1995), for example, shows how scientific claims and the construction of expertise straddle the divide between science and policy as alternate systems of authority. From my own study I see that negotiations and contestations among entrepreneurial, scientific, religious, and other sources of expertise affect classifications and legal constructions that in turn determine how body parts are understood legally, economically, and morally.

Wiederherstellung: *Putting It All Back Together*

Cultural understandings of the body and its use in technologies are situated within particular systems of power and specific historical, technological, geopolitical, and economic contexts. Within a liminal space and time in which organs are removed and then processed, bodily materials move out of the domain in which they are defined as a person's inviolable remains and into the medical pharmacopeia in the global economy. But within Germany, organs and tissues have attained a public presence that makes them simultaneously cultural and political symbols as well as technological objects.

The work practices and beliefs of those most directly involved, as well as the organizational and managerial practices of policymakers, legislators, journalists, and the public, interact to modify ideas and techniques surrounding the donor body and its parts. The nexus of participants and ideas is also affected by very old notions of animation in human bodily materials and the social and biological transitions that occur at death. Structures and institutions—education, religion, economic systems, laws—in part define the body and the meanings we have around it. Yet there is an interactivity between practices at these levels and practices at the hands-on level of dealing with the materiality of the body. Knowledge produced by the body itself, whether in the form of tacit and sensory experience or digital representation, is carried back to policy levels by participants (including surgeons, scientists, the public, the media, and others) who have ideas about appropriate treatment and use of body parts based on their experiences within cultures. These ideas include notions of what constitutes a violation to the body and to whom we give the authority to make such violations.

Organizational, economic, and technical innovations also adjudicate differences in the spheres of persons and commodities—as long as notions of rational medicine and technological progress are serving what appear to be agreed-upon norms. In this way, exchange and commerce can proceed while appearing to be consistent with western cultural interpretations of altruism and bodily integrity. This is particularly difficult in Germany, with its long history of ambivalence about the meaning of technological progress (Habermas 1988, Herf 1984, Bauman 1989).

There is a politics of recovery and redemption in the use of human materials. Recovering materials from bodies will help someone else recover, but the understandings of gain and loss are negotiated. Damaged bodies can be sites of redemption in which personal social identity and a sense of society as a whole—who "we" are—can be reinforced. For Germany, the politics of redemption involve restoring the reputation of German medicine and balancing the competing values of protection of individuals with the welfare of society.

The final form of the new law regarding the recovery and use of human material may appear to be little different from laws in many other countries, simply legitimizing the "business as usual" of organizing and practicing procurement. Nevertheless, the processes and people involved in negotiating the law kept several histories clearly in mind: a values-based constitution, links of governance and geography, and the specter of disastrous social engineering projects.

In its final form, the law includes provisions for the definition of brain death, permission to remove materials, and punishment for commercial sales of body parts. It states that families must be asked for permission to donate materials.[6] At the same time, the law and the debates surrounding its passage have reestablished the state as the site where the rights and

protection of the people are determined as well as understandings of inviolability, moving decisions out of the private domain of patients, families, and
physicians. Still, the claim to authority of medicine and medical expertise
in determining the end of life and the proper and respectful disposal of the
dead is supported by specific provisions about the medical criteria involved
in determining the point of death and choice of recipients.

Passing the law and setting up official channels and organizations to ex-
ecute its provisions is a public way to demonstrate that everything is under
control. Through its act of intervention, the state has exercised its role of
appearing to contain and discipline medicine. Medicine, in turn, has taken
advantage of the public nature of the debates surrounding the use of human bodies to display its rules, procedures, and protocols as being consistent with respect for persons while being based on universal scientific
norms. Thus, German medicine reestablishes itself as a credible steward
of German public health and attaching itself to international scientific efforts. At the bedside, German procurement practices are strongly affected
by the need to preserve an image of not violating the dead.

These are instrumental means of power. In the late twentieth century,
science, technology, and modern rationalized capitalism have been brought
together in ways that reshape social order. But the forms are not consistent and often contradictory. By focusing on core medical practices, I have
attempted to show the interactivity among institutional-level elements, local-
level practices, and the materiality of the body through which such
reorderings occur.

Appendix: Donation Rates and Public Opinion about Donation

In Germany, the number of organs and tissues voluntarily donated by families of brain-dead patients has steadily decreased in the 1990s. This contrasts with other European countries and the United States, where rates are either stable or rising. Table A.1 shows that in 1994 the rate in Germany dropped 25 percent (Eurotransplant Foundation 1994).

The number of donors reported by the Deutsche Stiftung für Organspende shows only a 12.6 percent decrease in the rate of donation in 1994, much smaller than the numbers reported by Eurotransplant (Deutsches Stiftung für Organspende 1994). Yet estimates I made from individual centers in Germany suggest an even greater decrease, ranging up to 35 percent in some clinics. The DSO reported 15.7 donors per million people in 1991 compared to an overall ET donor rate of 17.1 per million in the same year (Cohen 1994). The rate dropped to 12.7 donors per million by 1994, while overall ET rates grew slightly. Looked at in another way, estimates of the number of refusals to permit organ and tissue procurement increased from 21 percent in 1992 to 32 percent in 1993 (Deutsches Stiftung für Organspende 1994).[1]

Surveys by media and medical organizations have tried to gauge public attitudes toward voluntarily donating organs. The information in table A.2 was part of a survey that probed some deep concerns among the public that medical professionals had not been willing to admit.

_____ Table A.1 _____
Changes in Donation, Selected Countries, January–June 1994

Country	Percent Change
Germany	–25
United Kingdom	+4
Spain	+25
United States	+5

Source: Eurotransplant Foundation (1994); United Network for Organ Sharing (1994: 32).

A significant number of people surveyed appeared to mistrust the medical establishment and were either unsure or negative about giving permission to donate. Of those surveyed, 40.7 percent believed that organs are taken prematurely or were unsure whether or not they are taken too soon (Deutsche Stiftung für Organspende 1994). This survey suggested a significant east-west difference in attitudes and willingness to donate organs and tissues. There seems to be a steady increase of refusals in the west and a more stable and lower rate of refusal in the east.

Statistics for tissue donation are unreliable because a large proportion of tissue is used within the clinic where it is procured and not reported to outside organizations. Since different organizations and types of banks are involved, statistics and demographics regarding donor sources are kept in different ways. Nevertheless, some striking features differentiate the situation in Germany from other countries.

In interviews, German coordinators, pathologists, and physicians all stated that bone and skin are rarely procured. In fact, of the tissue registered and exchanged through BIS, none came from Germany between 1991 and 1994 (BioImplant Services 1992, 1993, 1994). Most respondents estimated that 85 to 90 percent of all skin used for burns and reconstructive surgery came from outside of Germany.

A public survey of willingness to donate tissue indicated that 70 percent of the public would be willing to donate a relative's corneas and heart valves. But when this was tested in practice by contacting relatives of newly dead patients, 66 percent refused (Schütt, Smit, and Duncker 1995). All the po-

——— *Table A.2* ———
Willingness to Donate Organs, Germany (in percent)

		West	East
Would you agree to donate your organs?	Yes	48	32
	No	21	22
	Not sure	31	46
I am not sure that doctors will handle my relative in the same way if he/she is a potential donor.	Agree	28	36
	Disagree	72	64

Source: Deutsche Stiftung für Organspende (1994).

tential donors were older patients with prolonged hospital stays, so refusals were not due to the shock of a sudden death, nor was there doubt that the patient was dead, as with brain-dead donors. Exacerbating the public's reluctance to donate tissue was reluctance from the coordinators themselves to request permission for tissue donation, much less make the necessary arrangements for procurement.

Notes

Unless otherwise noted, all translations are mine. Citations from my own field notes are abbreviated as "f.n." Occasionally I have edited the field notes to smooth out infelicities of translation or expression. Any field notes cited without specific months refer to comments made frequently by more than one respondent.

One Introduction

1. Examples include Clark (1993), Hirschauer (1991), Lock (1995), and Turner (1987, 1992).
2. Early contributions include Barley (1988), Jennett (1985), Koenig (1988), Plough (1981, 1986), and Reiser (1978).
3. Examples include Casper and Berg (1995); Downey, Dumit, and Williams (1995); and Latour (1987). See Basalmo (1992) for body alterations and Haraway (1991) for the implications thereof. Casper (1998), Dumit (1997), Hogle (1993, 1995c), Heath (1998), and Rapp (1988) have done ethnographic work that identifies various actors involved in changing constructions of the body.
4. See Franklin (1992), Haraway (1989, 1991), and Martin (1992, 1994). Marcus (1986) and Appadurai (1990) articulate the importance of multisited ethnography for reconceptualizing subjects in the particular global flows that exist at the end of the millennium.
5. See Braidotte (1989) and Stone (1992), among others.
6. On treatment of cadavers in organ donation, see Caplan (1984), Lamb (1985), and Youngner (1990). On the body as property, see Andrews (1986), Kimbrell (1993), Radin (1996), and Scott (1981).
7. Anderson's *Imagined Communities* (1983) is the cornerstone work in this regard, with important contributions from Hobsbawm and Ranger (1983). Later studies of specific processes in the overlapping of homogenizing and diversifying forces

include Appadurai (1990), Foster (1991), and Gupta and Ferguson (1992). See also Kahn (1992).

8. Harrington (1996), Harwood (1994), and Lenoir (1997) come to mind.

9. This has been particularly true of genetics research and work using fetal tissue, although restrictions have recently been quietly lifted and informal arrangements made to enable research to proceed. See Schlaes (1995) and Kahn (1992).

10. Gupta and Ferguson (1992) and Appadurai (1990) have convincingly argued against linking identity with geography, problematizing any discussion of national, ethnic, or other types of identity. Borneman (1992b) makes this case for the two Germanies. I wish to show how identities are multilayered in complex ways, cutting across professional, local or regional, historical, and political boundaries as well.

11. For expediency, I will use the names *East* and *West Germany* to talk about states belonging to the former two Germanies. My use of those names is not meant to perpetuate the "wall in the mind," as Germans call it, that maintains distinctions between two different countries.

12. The selection of political symbols and iconic events, heroes and narratives in the construction of national identity is discussed in Anderson (1983) and Hobsbawm and Ranger (1983), among others.

13. For example, the east's public health orientation allowed psychologists, homeopathic practitioners, and other therapists to participate in the insurance system. After unification, payment for these services was restricted. Eastern polyclinics were general rather than specialized, so there was little opportunity to form monopoly groups, a situation that changed with the disbanding of the former system. Powerful groups had interests in the reorganization process: pharmaceutical and medical manufacturing firms exert a strong influence on medical practice in the west, and insurance funds have more freedom to segregate funds based on risk groups. This was new to participants in the social medicine model in the east (Klinkmueller 1986, McKenzie 1990, D. Stone 1991).

14. Rather than finding a third way to blend the two systems, the entire East German medical system was reorganized. The polyclinics were dissolved, ambulatory care was privatized with new owners from the west who had credit and could purchase new equipment, and university medical professors and practitioners were let go in the process of examining professionals' records and ties to the Stasi. They were replaced by physicians from the west, and organizational and financing structures were changed.

15. After unification, physicians (like teachers, public officials, and others) were reviewed to determine if they had cooperated with the Communist government—in particular, if they had connections to the Stasi—that is, the Staatsicherheit: the secret police, who had a network of spies reporting on individual citizens. Most university physicians immediately lost their jobs either because of proof of compliance or simple accusations. Their experience is partly documented in Kruska (1994), "Fortschritt in der Medizin" (1994), and a series in *Deutsches Ärzteblatt* (Dauth 1994).

16. Today another form of dumping goes on in the east. Industries unable to obtain

permits or meet environmental standards or that lack public support in western sites find ample space and labor as well as strong financial incentives to go east. For example, a chemical company meant to be built in Lubeck was moved to Rostock when Green party activists demonstrated against it in Lubeck (f.n., July 1994). The Institute of Molecular Biotechnology built its new headquarters in Jena, along with 140 life science technology firms (Kahn 1995: 785). Gene technologies receive far less public resistance in the east, where a large pool of unemployed scientists are happy to have new jobs.

17. For example, one scenario described the use of a somewhat controversial technique to make a final determination in a patient whose brain-death diagnoses were unclear. Another scenario simply described physiological indicators indicating some difficulty, after which I asked how the physician would proceed.

18. See chapter 9 for a discussion of how the quality of materials is determined and how this affects exchange.

19. Changes in donation in the early 1990s varied among countries but generally showed an increase outside of Germany. Exceptions include Japan, where brain death has been an embattled concept, and France, where the national system was disbanded in a wave of scandals about management.

20. Examples of this approach to ethnography in the study of science, technology, and medicine include Heath (1998), Martin (1994), and Rapp (1988), among others.

21. My personal knowledge and background gave me the advantage of being familiar with hospital procedure. Previous experience in clinical medical technology was enormously helpful in understanding and critiquing the setting but was also key to gaining access to clinical areas, where social scientists are often unwelcome. I am extremely grateful to participants for their acceptance of me and for respecting my social science as well as my clinical perspective.

Part I

1. For example, body searches, including X rays and rectal exams, violate an individual's bodily boundaries, but a public interest in law enforcement can be construed as outweighing the individual's right to bodily privacy. Likewise, materials can be forcibly removed from criminal suspects. Tissue samples are often kept after surgery or biopsy and used for further study or processed into highly profitable products. These are the new sources and forms of power that infiltrate social life.

Two   Animation and Regeneration

1. Temple imagery appears, for example, in the verse: "Do you not know that your body is a temple of the Holy Spirit who is in you, whom you have from God and that you are not your own? . . . therefore glorify God in your body" (I Corinthians 6:19–20). The question of sanctity usually arises in debates about commercial uses of the body. Thus far, the courts have been unable to resolve these issues. In a now classic court case, a judge responded to the idea of considering a

plaintiff's bodily cells as commercial property in this way: "Plaintiff [has asked us to regard] the human vessel—the single most venerated and protected subject in any civilized society—as equal with the basest commercial commodity. He urges us to commingle the sacred with the profane. He asks much" (Justice Arabian in *Moore v. Regents of the University of California,* 793 P.2d 479, 497 [1990]). Legal debates over whether the body can be considered to be ownable property separable from the person are discussed in "Note, The Sale of Human Body Parts," *Michigan Law Review* 72 (1974): 1182, 1241.

2. I do not claim to be the first to note the similarities between contemporary and historical uses of the body. For example, Rabinow (1992b) draws the connection between cellular technologies and questions of bodily fragmentation unresolved since antiquity. Since I wrote the first drafts of this chapter, Youngner, Fox, and O'Connell (1996) have edited a volume that includes chapters on the history of dissection as well as myths and stories about the use of body parts through time, relating these topics to current ethical issues in transplant medicine.

3. To contextualize the discussion, two notes regarding information sources are necessary. First, the primary sources for conclusions about medieval and renaissance beliefs about the body at death are documents and official pronouncements from educated ecclesiastical figures. Thus, most information comes from the perspective of Judeo-Christian traditions (with an emphasis on the Christian). Nevertheless, popular beliefs about the body were strongly influenced by pagan rituals and beliefs through the seventh and eighth centuries. Funerary practices and treatment of the dead likely incorporated many of these beliefs, despite what official church documents state. This is particularly evident in the history of blood cults in Germany, which had pagan roots but were easily incorporated into Christian mythology (Ankert 1918, Linke 1986, Strack 1909).

   Second, assuming religious beliefs to be homogenous, historians have tended to generalize the effects of religious practices across all of Europe. There is some evidence to suggest, however, that beliefs about the nature of the body at death were similar across France, Belgium, and what is now Germany and that they varied in significant ways from cultural practices in southern and eastern Europe. In northern regions, including what is now Germany, ideas from Scandinavian and Slavic regions would likely have been introduced through immigration and trade.

   There is a great deal of information about views of the body at death between the tenth and the nineteenth centuries in France, Britain, and Italy. There is comparatively little material specific to Germany, even by German historians. This is due in part to the fact that what is now Germany was still a collection of small states within the Holy Roman Empire. Historians have focused on places where material may have been more readily available rather than on the centers of German medicine, which did not become prominent until later.

4. Kramer (1996) beautifully describes commemoration as a way of being able to create distance from active mourning.

5. While this was official church eschatology, treatises from pagan critics and ordinary congregations found it to be disgusting: who would want to have back

their used and putrid corpse? But it seems that more than body bits remained intact. Frescoes and paintings throughout Europe indicate that social status was retained at resurrection as well, judging by the manner of dress and goods that people carried with them.

6. Bynum adds that popular iconography often depicted hell as digestion and the gates of hell as a mouth. Likewise, there are numerous images of bodies being regurgitated whole from animals and body parts reassembling into wholes at the day of judgment. See also Binski (1996). Interestingly, a number of media articles discussing organ and tissue transplantation evoke themes of cannibalism (Emmrich 1994a).

7. See, for example, Ariès (1981), Foucault (1975, 1979), Richardson (1989), Rupp (1992), and Turner (1987), among others.

8. This is, of course, a highly simplified and abbreviated explanation of the transformation in understanding the body and the rise of clinical medicine. For more detailed discussions, see Foucault (1975, 1979) and Turner (1987, 1992).

9. Average pay for rural labor was about nine shillings per week during the eighteenth and early nineteenth centuries. A resurrectionist could get far more than that per exhumed or stolen body, and rare specimens for anatomical collections were worth several hundred British pounds. The easy means of income was an attractive alternative for some working-class people, especially those who were already socially marginal (Richardson 1989).

10. According to Richardson (1989: 90), the protests were unlike similar ones over economic wrongs such as price increases for food, the introduction of technology that eliminated jobs, or trespasses against morality such as adultery. In such cases, retribution involved burning effigies or circulating jokes and stories to regulate social behavior. She suggests that the poor recognized that it was mostly other poor who were victims and were thus reacting to a sense of class betrayal. The riots and demonstrations were a way of expressing feelings of anger and injustice that they could not express in other ways.

11. Gibbeting, flaying, and other total-body destruction techniques were also favored ways of dealing with enemies' bodies among both Catholics and Protestants in the religious battles following the Thirty Years' War.

12. The liquid was not only a remedy for a variety of serious illnesses but was reputed to be a diagnostic agent when mixed with the blood of a sick person—another example of the usefulness of body remains in producing scientific knowledge.

Three   Embodying National Identity

1. A great deal has been written about the unity of nationalism and Völkisch ideology, social hygiene, and eugenics in early twentieth-century Germany as well as the reconceptualization of German society. See, for example, Herf (1984); Mosse (1964/1981); Proctor (1988); Weindling (1989); and Weingart, Kroll, and Bayertz (1988).

2. In Germany today, cultural anthropologists (the American term) are called eth-

nologists. The word *anthropologist* refers to a physical or biological anthropologist who researches genetics, evolution, or related topics. This is an important distinction because the term *anthropology* is still often associated with racial hygiene programs. Physical and biological anthropologists in contemporary Germany are largely relegated to medical schools, but ethnologists distance themselves as much as possible from that work.

3. Brubaker (1992) notes the difference in the way in which German citizenship was differentially defined compared to citizenship in other countries, such as France. German citizenship, he argues, was based on blood descent and a sense of cultural and racial community as contrasted to French citizenship, which was framed around central political values and a defined sense of territory. Dumont (1986) has made similar comparisons, saying that France was a collective of individuals while the German nation was like a collective individual.

4. Metaphors of penetration and infection predate and invert Martin's (1992, 1994) and Haraway's (1989) suggestions that the use of military and political metaphors to explain bodily processes is a late capitalist phenomenon. In the German case, preventing infection and invasion of bodily boundaries was a metaphor for political—and eventually military—solutions to social problems rather than the other way around.

5. In Germany it was necessary to conduct a certain amount of research before being designated a physician. This is still true today. Students can finish medical school and practice medicine to a limited extent without research, but one has far less prestige and less career opportunity without this Ph.D. equivalent. A *Habilitation* is similar to a postdoctoral research appointment and is required for anyone planning to pursue an academic career. (The most prestigious posts are in university clinics.)

6. Extensive discussion of such experiments can be found in Lifton (1986), Mitscherlich (1949), and Pross and Aly (1989).

7. For more about the effects on contemporary bioethics, see Annas and Grodin (1992) and Kater (1987).

8. Lifton (1986) reports that about 46 percent of physicians were members of the National Socialist party. Other physicians I spoke to were trained by those who taught during the Nazi era. After the war, the surviving chief physicians in high academic positions were forced to leave their jobs. But the tremendous loss of life and the relatively small number of qualified physicians who were not party members meant that there was no one to replace them. Most of these faculty physicians eventually returned and continued their research and teaching.

9. Controversies about coming to terms with the past in a way that might normalize it erupted in a debate over the role and use of history. For coverage of this *Historikerstreit,* see the special issue of *New German Critique* (Spring–Summer 1988), in particular the articles by Habermas and Markovits. Regarding management of the past, see Czaplicka (1995), Huyssen (1995), Judt (1992), Kaes (1989), and Maier (1988).

Four   Culture, Technology, and the Law

1. Article II (2) ironically uses the word *eingriffen* for "interfere" or "intervene." This same word also means "surgical operation."
2. The following discussion is based primarily on Kommers (1995) but also developed from conversations with lawyers and a sociologist of law in Germany.
3. The law is based on many principles from the 1871 Bismarkian and Weimar constitutions, wedding a liberal Rechtsstaat (a state based on fixed and general laws) to the social welfare state.
4. Abortion is no longer punishable under criminal codes. It is not supported by federal welfare or insurance sources, but a woman can obtain an abortion if her pregnancy is life threatening. Still, she must find a physician willing to perform it (impossible in Catholic strongholds such as Bavaria) and undergo extensive counseling beforehand. Many women simply cross the border into the Netherlands.
5. Turner (1992) calls our attention to the distinction between Körper as the objective-instrumental body and Leib as the subjective-animate body, which figures into phenomenological studies of subjective bodily experiences.
6. Postmortem maternal ventilation refers to cases of brain-dead pregnant women who are kept on artificial support to sustain the fetus in hopes of saving its life. Note the use of *mother* rather than *woman,* which declares her role—and the role of her body—in this setting (see chapter 5).
7. This is not intended to be a detailed discussion of brain death. For background and history, see Rothman (1991). Gervais (1996) provides a useful discussion of various philosophical stances, including a biological defense (Becker 1975), ontological arguments (Lamb 1985), and moral arguments favoring a broader definition of death (Veatch 1976) or rejecting brain death as equivalent to death (Jonas 1974). For cultural beliefs in Japan affecting the use of this legal construction of death, see Lock and Honde (1990), Lock (1995), and Ohnuki-Tierney (1994). For cultural beliefs in the United States, see Hogle (1993).
8. Gesetzblatt der Deutschen Demokratischen Republik, Teil I Nr. 32 (August 6, 1975). The copy of the law was marked *ausgesondert,* indicating that it was not meant to be public, but most of the files regarding this and other defunct laws are now accessible.
9. Historical and geographical influences are evident in this case. Germany existed for centuries as a loosely bound collection of independent states; there was little history of centralized control until National Socialism. After the defeat of Nazism, institutions and governmental authority were intentionally returned to the regional and local levels to avoid the dangers of centralized control.
10. CDU members used language that made the state-versus-individual claim explicit. This language was echoed in headlines such as "Does the body belong to society?" (Emmrich 1994b) and "The state as organ dealer" (Graupner 1994).
11. See Singer (1994) about the debates over rationing neonatal care in Germany.
12. Of course, other economic and political interests may also be involved. See, for example, Richard Evans's (1987) fascinating account of the handling of an epidemic in Hamburg. In this particular case, such interests were at odds with

public health concerns during decisions about whether to quarantine the city and close the port to trade.

13. Some would argue that prenatal testing, selective abortion, and genetic testing with the admonition not to reproduce defective genes are similar quarantining actions, if not outright duplications of eugenics programs.

14. For now, access to tissue in the United States is based on a donation system, relying on notions of altruism and gift giving. Access has been boosted by public rulings such as the 1986 Budget Reconciliation Act, which requires hospitals to request organs and tissues from families of brain-dead patients (PL 99–509 [1986]). Various proposals have been made to allow unrestricted access to cadaver materials (Hansmann 1989, Blumstein 1989).

15. Jasanoff (1995) eloquently discusses how questions of individual liberty and social needs are framed, using the examples of persistent vegetative states and severely handicapped newborns.

Five Bodies, Sciences, and the State

1. The legal limit for abortion is twelve weeks.

2. See, for example, *Frankfurter Rundschau* (1992), *Der Spiegel* (1992), *Deutsches Ärzteblatt* (1993), and Wuermeling (1992).

3. Eventually an aunt was given responsibility for the woman, keeping the interests of fetus and woman distinct.

4. The criterion for brain-death declaration in Germany appears in *Deutsches Ärzteblatt* (1991). Diagnostic techniques appear in Haupt et al. (1993).

5. Many of the articles written about the case focused on questions of what constituted quality of life for the fetus. The woman was practically invisible in both the popular media and in medical accounts; when she did appear, she was referred to as a corpse. The exceptions were either articles that highlighted the bizarre circumstances (*Der Spiegel* 1992) or those written from feminist perspectives. The latter raised the question of dignity and the right to die and the use of women's bodies as birth machines (*Tageszeitung* 1992). Regarding postmortem maternal ventilation, see Hartouni (1991) and Murphy (1989).

6. In my own observations and reviews of protocols, brain-death declaration criteria and procedures were at least as thorough as those in the west—sometimes even more stringent, requiring the agreement of three unrelated physicians rather than two.

7. Organs, in this case, refer primarily to kidneys, although heart transplantation was performed to a limited extent in Berlin.

8. German research is partially funded by the National Highway Traffic Safety Administration in the United States. The Centers for Disease Control in Atlanta fund similar research in the United States.

9. He bases this claim on the fact that many organ donors are accident victims or suicides.

10. Compare to the United States, which primarily has positive media coverage of organ donation.

11. See Gilman (1991) on the depiction of Jews, Proctor (1988) and Linke (1986) on representation of non-Aryan bodies. See also the films of Leni Riefenstahl.

Part II

1. See, for example, Hacking (1992) and Pickering (1992) for the theory of practice as the creative work of bringing together elements necessary to accomplish scientific tasks. The essays in Bijker, Hughes, and Pinch (1987) discuss the social shaping of technologies, including elements that contribute to the stability (or lack thereof) of forms that technologies take. Hess (1996) extends the critical and cultural analysis of knowledge making in science to include important considerations of race and gender.
2. Most states now have required request and reporting rules; that is, a hospital must report a potential donor to the OPO, and there must be a procedure in place for approaching the family about donation. Compliance with these rules is part of the accreditation process mandated by the Joint Commission on Accreditation of Health Organizations (f.n., March 1992; Rettig 1989).
3. In the United States, these coordinators are usually registered nurses with considerable intensive care experience. There are also transplant coordinators based inside transplant centers who deal with organ recipients only. In this book, I do not discuss U.S. transplant coordinators in detail.
4. Brief overviews of the official version of the German system can be found in Feuerstein (1996) and Schutt, Smit, and Schroeder (1992).
5. Not everyone gets registered. The decision about acceptance varies greatly by transplant center, depending on the center's selection criteria and committee decisions. If accepted, a potential recipient pays a registration fee to the network organization (here, UNOS or ET).
6. Often families give permission for only one organ, or some organs may be too damaged to use. In most cases, U.S. coordinators ask families for several organs and/or tissues. In Germany, tissues are rarely requested and rarely retrieved. If they are used, they involve very little intervention from Koordinatoren.
7. The decision to ship an organ takes into consideration several factors. Surgeons I interviewed explained that kidneys are "tough" and "can take more abuse" than other organs. Heart and liver surgeons prefer to see the condition of the organ in situ to determine if it has too much fatty tissue or is otherwise a so-called "low-quality" organ. I have heard similar comments throughout both the United States and Germany.

Six   Organizing Procurement

1. This refers to cadaver organs only; living donors were arranged for differently. Tissues came from genetically related individuals, meaning fewer problems of tissue rejection.
2. If antigens are present in the donor and there are corresponding antigens in the potential recipient or host, or if there is a corresponding absence of the antigens, there will be no antibodies against the antigens to cause a reaction.

3. The system is used primarily for kidneys; there is some controversy among transplant researchers about application to other organs. Also, additional factors such as waiting time on the list are considered in many programs.

   Interestingly, HLA antigens are used in various ways in allocation debates. Immunologists and transplanters argue that various races have statistically different arrays of these genetically determined antigens and are thus less likely to be a good match for members of other races. This is offered as an explanation for the unequal proportion of persons of color on waiting lists who actually get organs compared with white patients who receive transplants. Because persons of color do not donate enough organs, the argument goes, there are not enough good matches for people of the same racial group. The solution often proposed is to target donation promotion campaigns at these ethnic groups rather than find alternative solutions to the matching problem (cf. Barger et al. 1992, Parham 1993, Thompson 1995). This has the effect of reifying racial categories, despite the fact that there is more genetic variation within groups than between them.

4. I dislike making the distinction between "medical" and "nonmedical" because any work involved in medicine is medical work. Medicine is, after all, practiced as much over the telephone and the fax line as it is by the bedside. My point, however, is to underscore the fact that far more goes on to produce exchangeable tissues than what goes on inside the operating room. The German physicians I spoke to certainly did distinguish between nonmedical and medical work and personnel.

5. Braun and Joerges (1993) point out that first-order technical systems, particularly transport and communications, were essential for the expansion of organ exchange networks. Although I agree, I believe that far more complex cultural and economic reasons have pushed the course of transplantation technology.

6. Member countries included East Germany, Czechoslovakia, the Soviet Union, Hungary, Poland, and, interestingly, Cuba.

7. The United Kingdom, Luxembourg, and Spain also participate in meetings and occasionally exchange organs.

8. My experience, however, is limited to the United States and Europe.

9. The word *transparent* appears repeatedly in articles in the medical literature and in presentations to the public. It is meant to convey the idea that there is no mystique or mismanagement—that anyone can look in and understand what happens with brain-dead donors and their organs.

10. Exchange imbalances are closely tracked and recorded in annual meetings and publications as import and export balances, much like other trade goods.

11. Germany actually produced 55.3 percent of BIS donor hearts for valve processing in 1994, but about half each year are discarded due to procedural errors or morphology (see chapter 9) or for other reasons. Most of these donor hearts come from two major heart clinics that donate hearts discarded from transplant procedures ("domino" hearts).

12. Competition among clinics is brought into the political arena when local governments mandate that certain procedures can be done at some clinics and not

others. This is particularly visible in Berlin, which existed previously as two cities.

13. After I finished my research, this organization split into two groups, one of which immediately disbanded. The move was intended to remove the old guard and install a new power core.

14. In the United States, arrangements are made for the OPO to pay for all procurement expenses from the moment of formal brain-death declaration through the removal procedure. The transplanting center must then purchase the organ from the OPO. These costs, plus surgeon fees and patient care and hospital fees, are reimbursed by Medicare (kidneys) or insurance payers. The prices vary by organ and are exclusive of other costs. The politics and economics of organ and services pricing in the United States are beyond the scope of this book. For more information, see Rettig (1989) and Prottas (1985), among others.

15. Coordinators often refer to the DSO as a *Wasserkopf,* meaning the bureaucratic, overgrown head of the organization. The word literally means the enlarged head of a child born with "water on the brain" (hydrocephalus).

16. The one exception was the official mantra that all transactions in the exchange of human organs are put through Eurotransplant.

17. The interested reader can find these trade routes in Baume (1969), Bechtel (1952), and Schildhauer (1988).

18. Since the time of this study, cooperation seems to have fallen apart. According to follow-up reports from respondents, this is largely because of the imbalance of organs, especially kidneys, between east and west.

19. The 1975 East German Transplant Law states that Friedrichshain in Berlin is the site of central coordination.

20. Many people did not have phones because lines were not as extensive as they were in the west. Many others did not want phones because they were a primary means of information for the Stasi.

21. This is written into guidelines of professional organizations, which state that human material can be removed if ethically justified or if there is an urgent need. The Transplantationskodex written by the Arbeitsgemeinschaft der Transplantationszentren in West Germany (consisting primarily of transplant surgeons) makes general recommendations for procuring organs from living and dead donors, tissue typing, and exchanging organs. It forbids selling organs for profit. After the cadaver tissue removal scandals in 1993, warnings were issued to hospitals not to allow sales, but specific rules and wordings varied by city and region.

Seven   Local Practice

1. The term *coordinator* usually refers to the physician, but in some centers it refers to an administrative worker.

2. The European Transplant Coordinator Organization (ETCO) is a pan-European group that attempts to set standards for practice and promote this work as a profession. The National Association of Transplant Coordinators (NATCO) is the U.S. sister organization. There are 250 members of ETCO in Europe (with a

population of 300 million) and 1,600 members in the United States (with a population of 255 million).

3. In cases of accidental death or suspected homicide, the coroner will inspect the body for evidence. This often leads to disputes about whether or not a procurement procedure may be done, when, and what parts of the body cannot be touched. There are also frequent questions about jurisdiction, especially if the death occurred in a place different from where the body was taken for treatment. Such battles for control (ownership?) of the body are a fascinating area for future research on the nexus of legal, medical, religious, and other social constructions of the good of society, the furthering of knowledge, and allowable uses of the body.

4. Transplant teams in the United States and Germany will occasionally remove additional organs and ship them to the center listing the recipient who has been matched through UNOS or ET. This is most common with kidneys. Livers are less often shipped, especially in Germany, where they are closely inspected by the implanting team. Hearts are never shipped.

5. Since my research was concerned with procurement rather than transplant practices, I have not analyzed distribution decisions related to organ recipients. Volker Schmidt (1996), however, has covered these issues in detail. He interviewed a number of transplant surgeons, finding very arbitrary justifications for allowing patients onto the waiting list. According to Schmidt, among the factors used were the patient's social responsibility, age, and lifestyle.

6. For hearts and livers, the urgency category of the recipient (as judged by the transplant surgeon) is taken into account as well as the number of procedures performed during the previous year by the transplant center where the patient is registered. In Germany at the time of my research, livers were center-driven, except for a category of high-urgency patients. Hearts were patient-driven, although there have been several attempts to make them center-driven.

7. To augment the ET system, some surgeons and coordinators have also formed regional consortiums with their own pooled list of waiting patients (see chapter 6).

8. For example, so-called "designer" monoclonal antibodies will be donor-specific. One approach gets the host T-cells to "learn" not to reject the new tissue, and another creates chimeras between donor and recipient cells, fooling the host immune system into accepting them. See also the discussion about preservatives in chapter 8.

9. Transplantation is fully reimbursed by the German insurance system, and fees are not controlled. Transplant recipients are required to return to the same transplant center (often to an outpatient clinic owned by transplant surgeons) for follow-up visits for at least a year. Several respondents told me that this is where the most income is made, although I was unable to document that information in hospital records.

10. The coordinator used the word *hautnah* (skin-close) to describe the feeling of having something too near or too personal.

Eight Converting Human Materials

1. Examples of observations of such interactions can be found in Clarke and Fujimura (1992), Clause (1993), and Kohler (1994), among others.
2. The comparison with abortion may trouble some readers: the existence of "person" before the point of removal is highly contested, and the fetus never lived as a separate entity apart from the woman's body. My point here, however, is to find another situation in which categories of person and thing are carefully constructed to allow certain actions and procedures.
3. This trend is apparent in many countries, with varying degrees of controversy. Essentially, donors with certain kinds of cancers (or histories of) or other conditions are now considered eligible for donation, causing understandable concern about spreading the disease and malfunction of the organ due to disease. The counterargument, however, (at least in the United States) is that if the recipient survives long enough to experience problems, she can always be fixed by other treatments and technologies or by retransplanting the malfunctioning organ.
4. At the same time, I was told that there is no discrimination against organ recipients based on ethnicity or national origin. In fact, I was led into a room where a recipients' self-help group was being conducted. The coordinator pointed at a Turkish man and said loudly, "See, we do give organs to other races. We don't just give them to Germans" (f.n., January 1994).
5. Travel to certain countries might raise questions about parasites or infection; residents of long-term care facilities are often exposed to tuberculosis and other infections; and tattooing instruments, if not properly disinfected, can transmit microorganisms such as HIV.
6. There is usually one central venous line, a Swan-Ganz line, an arterial line, as well as peripheral venous lines. As one respondent said, adding a fifth, "you never can have too many lines."
7. Some would say that the person lives on in the organs themselves. Sharp (1995), for example, has collected data that suggest a strong belief among donor families and organ recipients that the organ continues to carry an essence of the donor's person.
8. For example, in one case I observed, a donor's fiancée wanted to attempt to have sperm removed so she could bear his child. In another, a donor's common-law partner had no legal access to the donor's bank account or personal records; the case was held for two days until she could get power of attorney. The donor was diagnosed as brain dead on a Saturday and legally declared dead after the legal matter was settled Monday evening.
9. The term *resuscitation* is also applied to fluid replacement.
10. For example, one effect of brain death on the liver is that Kupffer cells are activated, accompanied by the release of tissue necrosis factors and interleukins, which break down liver sinus cells. In animal experiments, researchers have injected gadolinium chloride into donors to block this activity; two days later organs were removed and transplanted (Motoyama et al. 1995). See also Novitzky, Cooper, Rose, and Reichert (1987); Korb et al. (1989); and Wechsler (1989).

11. A cannula is a plastic tube inserted into the body, usually to drain fluids.

12. This is not a gown that would normally protect personnel from acquiring or spreading infectious agents between patients. That type of gown would be disposed of after a procedure. Instead, the gown remains hanging inside the room and is aimed at protecting patients from outside infections. The gown also creates another barrier between personnel and the dead.

13. Preservation chemicals are used, however, once the materials are removed from the body. Interestingly, two respondents in different clinics referred to this as *die Lagerung* (storage). The same word is used for marinades or seasoning, such as those for meat.

14. See, for example, Cambrosio and Keating (1988), Berg (1997), Clarke (1998), Fujimura (1987), and Knorr-Cetina (1981), among others.

15. In many ways this is parallel to fetal surgery or postmortem maternal ventilation, in which the woman's body becomes the protective environment that allows the fetus to exist while hindering access to and care for the fetus as a patient.

Nine   The Right Theraputic Tools

1. This chapter graphically describes the removal of organs and tissues from the body, which may disturb some readers. I have attempted to describe the technical content of the work in a straightforward way, applying the notion of anthropological strangeness without trying to sensationalize the topic.

2. The theme of sacrifice for others is consistent in organ donation literature, which often refers to the biblical lessons of "laying down one's life for one's friends" and "dying so that others may live," even though donors do not intentionally die for this purpose. Rather, these views reinforce the idea that good can come from a tragic death. The film *Jesus of Montreal* expands on this theme. See also Hogle (1996).

3. See Flye (1995: 48–60) for a generalized description of the technical aspects of the procedure.

4. This incident also shows the hierarchical roles in the operating room. Although everyone was clearly disturbed, no one attempted to contradict or stop the surgeon. The jokes were probably an indirect way of registering disagreement.

5. While suspending the procedure was difficult for everyone else, it was an extraordinary opportunity for me. It allowed me a rare chance to speak to the anesthesiologist alone and to the OR nurses, most of whom had never experienced a procurement procedure before. They described a feeling of strangeness but were not horrified, as many writers have suggested (Striebel and Link 1993). One reason why the coordinator in charge made another attempt to use the heart was "so the staff could have a positive first experience." That is, he wanted the staff to feel that their efforts were productive—that all this was not just for kidneys.

6. This is about $40,000 and $200, respectively.

7. Warm ischemic time is counted from cross-clamp to the time when the organ is cooled. Cold ischemic time is the duration of cold preservation. These times are

recorded on all forms because practitioners believe that length of ischemic time affects subsequent organ function.

8. Indeed, in the OPO I studied in the United States, staffing was changing to employ nonmedical personnel as the primary transmitters of donor data to transplant centers.

9. This is not to suggest that a homogeneous national characteristic can be generalized. Still, in many observations of numerous everyday activities, one sees certain patterns emerge.

10. The irony, of course, is that this work, now reserved for the most elite in the German medical hierarchy, was once the territory of barber-surgeons, historically very low-status practitioners.

11. Shapin (1994: 381) has discussed the way that tacit and direct knowledge is valued, suggesting that it is dependent on the moral nature of social relations in the workplace. Although he refers to the relations of technicians and scientists in an experimental setting, there is a parallel to the valuing of various types of knowledge within the social relations of organ procurement.

12. U.S. insurers have not fully incorporated liver transplantation into payment schemes because it is a newer and more costly procedure than other kinds of transplantation and procedures can only be done at certified centers. Transplant centers are certified based on the frequency of procedures they perform. This is intended to measure expertise.

13. This will likely change in the next few years of health care reform as services are rationed to clinics that do the greatest number of certain procedures.

14. Graft survival is defined as how long the organ or tissue survives in the host before it fails due to immunological reaction or other complications. Patient survival is the life span of the transplanted patient after receiving the transplant.

15. The tissue becomes harder (cell membranes become rigid), and damage occurs when the organ is reperfused. The mitochondria release ATP; oxygen escapes and is reduced to water in an uncontrolled manner, giving rise to free oxygen radicals that damage tissue. Reperfusion is considered to be more detrimental than ischemic time when there is no blood circulation or oxygenation (Thaw 1994).

Ten Conclusions

1. The Gene Law of 1990 is one of the world's most comprehensive laws regulating the use of recombinant DNA technology. It requires a series of public hearings and examinations by enforcement officials for laboratories to create, exchange, or use genetically altered materials (Kahn 1992).

2. The manner of allocation and acquisition are discussed in chapter 6. See also Volker Schmidt (1996) for a well-documented study of how medical professionals in Germany make local decisions about allocation even in the face of standard medical criteria. For a similar view in the United States, see Hogle (1995b).

3. The sporting event is a national Olympics-like event that celebrates the success of transplant medicine. During my ethnographic research in a U.S. organ procurement organization, I observed annual memorial celebrations of various types,

ranging from a plaque with the donor's name to a mass memorial service held for all donors during the year. Procurement coordinators also often contacted donor families at the one-year anniversary of the donation.
4. Insightful summaries appear in Casper and Koenig (1996), Franklin (1995), and Martin (1998).
5. See also Hess (1996) for an excellent discussion of alternative knowledge. Marshall, Thomasma, and Daar (1996) study the clash of technological and economic exigencies with competing moral authorities. Their example is kidney brokering in India.
6. The debate over passage of the law lasted more than five hours, with most of that time taken up with the question of brain death.

Appendix

1. According to my observations, the numbers of refusals reflected in official reports are often considerably understated; families are never approached when there is any concern that they might react negatively or if a family physician or hospital neurologist may present a problem. No reason for refusal is recorded, and statistics are uneven because information is only voluntarily provided to organizations outside transplant centers.

Glossary

angiogram   an X ray of a vessel. Radiopaque material is injected so blockage can be seen.

BioImplant Services (BIS)   a not-for-profit organization that organizes tissue procurement activities for European countries, sponsors research, and conducts technical education programs.

cannula   a plastic tube inserted into the body to drain excess fluid.

computerized tomography (CAT)   radiographic examination of internal structures of the body.

Deutsche Stiftung für Organspende (DSO)   a not-for-profit organization founded by the Kuratorium für Hemodialyse in Germany that organizes organ procurement activities in some transplant centers.

echocardiogram   ultrasound test to determine movement patterns of the heart and heart valves. Results are displayed graphically.

Eurotransplant Foundation   a not-for-profit organization that organizes organ procurement and transplant activities, including the matching of information between donors and recipients. Member countries include the Netherlands, Germany, Austria, and Belgium.

explantation   removal of organs to be implanted in a transplant recipient (also called procurement).

German Democratic Republic (GDR)   East Germany before reunification.

herniation   the process of forming an abnormal protrusion. In brain herniation, tissue swells to such a point that function ceases.

human leukocytic antigens (HLA)   a set of antigens on the surface of white blood cells. The pattern of certain key antigens are used to characterize or "type" the tissue of the donor, and this type is matched as closely as possible to the potential recipient to prevent tissue rejection from antigen-antibody reactions. HLA matching is used primarily for kidney allocation.

ischemia   lack of blood flow in a body area, causing damage.

intravenous (IV)   refers to the introduction of fluids into the veins using a plastic tube.

Kuratorium für Hemodialyse (KfH)   a not-for-profit organization that manages dialysis centers throughout Germany. Principal participants are also active in kidney transplantation.

Leiche, Leichnam   cadaver.

mos teutonicus   medieval German custom of dividing parts of the corpse to bury in several locations.

organ procurement organization (OPO)   a not-for-profit organization in the United States that organizes organ procurement for a specified geographical region. OPOs contract their services through the United Network for Organ Sharing.

Pietätsempfinden   a sense of reverence, particularly in reference to the dead.

Scheintod   apparent death. In other words, the body appears to be dead but is still alive. This was a great concern in northern Europe between the thirteenth and seventeenth centuries.

spinal reflex   a reflex that causes muscles to contract, producing the effect of moving or twitching. This is often observed in severely brain-injured and brain-dead bodies.

Totenruhe   the peace of the dead.

Totensorgerecht   the right of family to care for the dead and make customary funeral arrangements.

United Network for Organ Sharing (UNOS)   the not-for-profit, federally contracted organization in the United States responsible for coordinating national organ procurement and transplant activities.

Widerspruchslösung   an East German law, no longer in effect, that allowed surgeons to remove organs and tissues for transplantation or research without permission from next of kin.

Bibliography

Akrich, Madeleine. 1992. "The De-Scription of Technical Objects." In *Shaping Technology/Building Society,* edited by Wiebe E. Bijker and John Law, 205–24. Cambridge: MIT Press.

Anderson, Benedict. 1983. *Imagined Communities.* New York: Verso.

Andrews, Lynn. 1986. "My Body, My Property." *Hastings Center Report* 16: 28–35.

Angstwurm, H. 1987. "Definition und Bestimmung des Hirntodes." *Intensivmedizin* 24: 395–99.

———. 1990. "Der Hirntod—ein sicheres Todeszeichen." *Wiener Medizinische Wochenschrift* 4: 112–16.

Ankert, Heinrich. 1918. "Menschenblut als Medizin." *Österreichische Zeitschrift für Volkskunde* 24: 131.

Annas, George, and Michael Grodin. 1992. *The Nazi Doctors and the Nuremberg Code.* New York: Oxford University Press.

Appadurai, Arjun. 1986. "Introduction: Commodities and the Politics of Value." In *The Social Life of Things,* edited by A. Appadurai, 3–63. New York: Cambridge University Press.

———. 1990. "Disjuncture and Difference in the Global Cultural Economy." *Public Culture* 2: 1–23.

Ariès, Philippe. 1981. *The Hour of Our Death.* New York: Oxford University Press.

Barger, B., T. Schoyer, S. Hudson, M. Deierkoi, et al. 1992. "The Impact of the UNOS Mandatory Sharing Policy on Recipients of the Black and White Races." *Transplantation* 53: 770–74.

Barley, Stephen. 1988. "The Social Construction of a Machine: Ritual, Superstition, Magical Thinking and Other Pragmatic Responses to Running a CT Scanner." In *Biomedicine Examined,* edited by Margaret Lock and Deborah Gordon, 497–540. Boston: Kluwer.

219

Basalmo, Anne. 1992. "On the Cutting Edge: Cosmetic Surgery and the Technological Production of the Gendered Body." *Camera Obscura* 258: 207–38.

Battaglia, Debbora. 1992. "The Body in the Gift: Memory and Forgetting in Sabarl Mortuary Exchange." *American Ethnologist* 19, no. 1: 3–18.

———. 1993. "At Play in the Fields (and Borders) of the Imaginary: Melanesian Transformations of Forgetting." *Cultural Anthropology* 8, no. 4: 430–42.

Baudrillard, Jean. 1993. *Symbolic Exchange and Death*. Thousand Oaks, Calif.: Sage.

Bauman, Zygmunt. 1989. *Modernity and the Holocaust*. New York: Polity.

———. 1992. *Mortality, Immortality and Other Life Strategies*. Stanford: Stanford University Press.

Baume, Franz. 1969. *Medieval Civilization in Germany, 800–1273*. New York: Praeger.

Bechtel, Heinrich. 1952. *Wirtschaftsgeschichte Deutschland*. Munich: Georg Callweg Verlag.

Becker, Lawrence. 1975. "Human Being: The Boundaries of the Concept." *Philosophy and Public Affairs* 4: 335–59.

Berg, Marc. 1997. *Rationalizing Medical Work: Decision Support Techniques and Medical Practices*. Cambridge: MIT Press.

Bergman, Anna, Gabriele Czarnowski, and Annegret Ehmann. 1989. "Menschen als Objekte humangenetischer Forschung und Politik im 20. Jahrhundert." In *Der Wert des Menschen*, edited by Christian Pross and Goetz Aly. Berlin: Ärtzekammer Berlin u. Bundeskammer.

Bijker, Wiebe E., Thomas Hughes, and Trevor Pinch, eds. 1987. *The Social Construction of Technological Systems: New Directions in the Sociology and History of Technology*. Cambridge: MIT Press.

Bild-Zeitung. 1993. "Was passiert mit mir nach meinem Tod?" November 25, pp. 1–2.

Binski, Paul. 1996. *Medieval Death: Ritual and Representation*. Ithaca, N.Y.: Cornell University Press.

BioImplant Services. 1992. *Annual Report*. Leiden.

———. 1993. *Annual Report*. Leiden.

———. 1994a. *Annual Report*. Leiden.

———. 1994b. Brochure. Leiden.

Birnbacher, D., H. Angstwurm, F. W. Eigler, and H. B. Wuermeling. 1993. "Der vollständige und endgültige Ausfall der Hirntätigkeit als Todeszeichen des Menschen—Anthropologischer Hintergrund." *Deutsches Ärzteblatt* 90: 2993–98.

Bloch, Maurice, and Jonathan Parry, eds. 1982. *Death and the Regeneration of Life*. New York: Cambridge University Press.

Blumstein, James. 1989. "Government's Role in Organ Transplantation Policy." *Journal of Health Politics, Policy, and Law* 14: 5–40.

Borneman, John. 1992a. *Belonging in the Two Berlins*. New York: Cambridge University Press.

———. 1992b. "State, Territory and Identity Formation in the Postwar Berlins, 1945–1989." *Cultural Anthropology* 7: 44–61.

Braidotte, Rosi. 1989. "Organs without Bodies." *Differences* 1, no. 1: 147–61.

Braun, Ingo, and Bernward Joerges. 1993. "How to Recombine Large Technical Systems: The Case of European Organ Transplantation." Occasional paper. Berlin: Wissenschaftszentrum für Sozialforschung Berlin.

Brautigam, Hans Harald. 1994. "Todlicher Streit." *Die Zeit,* July 8, p. 25.

Brown, Elizabeth. 1981. "Death and the Human Body in the Late Middle Ages: The Legislation of Boniface VII on the Division of Corpses." *Viator* 12: 221–70.

Brubaker, Rogers. 1992. *Citizenship and Nationhood in France and Germany.* Cambridge: Harvard University Press.

Bynum, Carolyn Walker. 1990. "Material Continuity, Personal Survival and the Resurrection of the Body: A Scholastic Discussion in Its Medieval and Modern Contexts." *History of Religions* 56: 51–83.

———. 1995a. *The Resurrection of the Body in Western Christianity, 200–1336.* New York: Columbia University Press.

———. 1995b "Why All the Fuss about the Body? A Medievalist's Perspective." *Critical Inquiry* 22: 1–33.

Cambrosio, Alberto, and Peter Keating. 1988. "Going Monoclonal: Art, Science and Magic in the Day-to-Day Use of Hybridoma Technology." *Social Problems* 35: 244–60.

Caplan, Arthur. 1984. "Ethical and Policy Issues in the Procurement of Cadaver Organs for Transplantation." *New England Journal of Medicine* 311, no. 15: 981–83.

———. 1992. "The Doctors' Trial and Analogies to the Holocaust in Contemporary Bioethical Debates." In *The Nazi Doctors and the Nuremberg Code,* edited by G. Annas and M. Grodin, 258–75. New York: Oxford University Press.

Casper, Monica. 1994. "At the Margins of Humanity: Fetal Positions in Science and Medicine." *Science, Technology, and Human Values* 19, no. 3: 307–23.

———. 1998. *The Making of the Unborn Patient: Medical Work and the Politics of Reproduction in Experimental Fetal Surgery, 1963–1993.* New Brunswick: Rutgers University Press.

Casper, Monica, and Marc Berg. 1995. "Constructivist Perspectives on Medical Work: Medical Practices and Science and Technology Studies." *Science, Technology, and Human Values* 20: 395–407.

Casper, Monica, and Barbara Koenig. 1996. "Reconfiguring Nature and Culture: Intersections of Medical Anthropology and Technoscience Studies." *Medical Anthropology Quarterly* 10: 523–36.

Clark, Margaret. 1993. "Medical Anthropology and the Redefining of Human Nature." *Human Organization* 52: 223–42.

Clarke, Adele. 1998. *Disciplining Reproduction: Modernity, American Life Sciences, and the "Problems of Sex."* Berkeley: University of California Press.

Clarke, Adele, and Joan Fujimura. 1992. "What Tools? Which Jobs? Why Right?" In *The Right Tools for the Job,* edited by Adele Clarke and Joan Fujimura, 3–44. Princeton: Princeton University Press.

Clarke, Adele, and Theresa Montini. 1993. "The Many Faces of RU486: Tales of Situated Knowledges and Contested Technologies." *Science, Technology, and Human Values* 18, no. 1: 42–78.

Clause, Bonnie. 1993. "The Wistar Rat As a Right Choice: Establishing Mammalian

Standards and the Ideal of a Standardized Mammal." *Journal of the History of Biology* 26: 329–49.

Clauss, L. F. 1936. *Rasse und Seele: eine Einführung in den Sinn der leiblichen Gestalt.* Munich: Lehrmann.

Cohen, Bernard. 1994. "Finding a Cure to Dramatic Falls in Organ Procurement." *Nephrology News and Issues/Europe* (July–August): 10–11.

Conklin, Beth. 1995. "Thus Are Our Bodies, Thus Was Our Custom: Mortuary Cannibalism in an Amazonian Society." *American Ethnologist* 22, no. 1: 75–101.

Council of Europe. 1994. *Convention for the Protection of Human Rights and Dignity with Regard to the Application of Biology and Medicine.* Strasbourg: Council of Europe.

Czaplicka, Jahn. 1995. "History, Aesthetics and Contemporary Commemorative Practice in Berlin." *New German Critique* 65: 155–87.

Daston, Lorraine. 1995. "Preternatural Philosophy." Paper presented at a meeting of the Max Planck Institute for the History of Science, Berlin, September 19.

Dauth, Sabine. 1994. "Manchmal nahm das Interview die Form einer Debatte an." *Deutsches Ärzteblatt* 91, no. 19: C869–70.

de Jong, I. J., and J. Kranenburg. 1995. "Standard Treatment Organ Donor Protocol Prevents Circulatory Instability after Brain Death." In *Current Aspects and Concepts of Nursing, Coordination, Bridging and Rehabilitation in Organ Transplantation,* edited by M. M. Koerner and R. Koerfer, 43–48. New York: Elsevier.

Der Spiegel. 1992. "Leben in der Leiche." 43: 320–327.

———. 1993a. "Geplündert ins Grab." 39: 68–80.

———. 1993b. "Rammbock in die Flanke." 38: 210–12.

———. 1993c. "Wem gehört eine Leiche?" 39: 77.

———. 1994a. "Gedränge an der Leiche." 39: 206–10.

———. 1994b. "0,2 Prozent einer Leiche." 39: 142–45.

———. 1994c. "Allgemeines Rätsel." 29: 38.

———. 1995a. "Häßliche Grauzone." 50: 87–88.

———. 1995b. "Sollen wir den Embryo verbrennen?" 40: 223.

Deutsches Ärzteblatt. 1991. "Kriterien des Hirntodes." 88: B2855–60.

———. 1993. "Rettung des Erlanger Babys weder geboten noch verboten." 90: C65–66.

———. 1994. "Abort oder Totgeburt: ein schmaler Grat." 91, no. 8: 376.

Deutsche Stiftung für Organspende. 1992. *Jahresbericht.* Neu-Isenburg.

———. 1993. *Jahresbericht.* Neu-Isenburg.

———. 1994. *Jahresbericht.* Neu-Isenburg.

Die Woche. 1994a. "Nur über meine Leiche." June 23, p. 18.

———. 1994b. "Wann ist der Mensch tot genug?" June 27, p. 28.

Dölger, F. 1926. *Antike und Christentum: Kulture und religiose Geschichte.* Munich: Verlag der Bayerische Akademie der Wissenschaften.

Downey, Gary, Joe Dumit, and Sarah Williams. 1995. "Cyborg Anthropology." In *The Cyborg Handbook,* edited by Chris Gray, 341–46. New York: Routledge.

Dumit, Joe. 1997. "A Digital Image of the Category of the Person: PET Scanning and Objective Self-Fashioning." In *Cyborgs and Citadels: Anthropological Investi-*

gations in Emerging Sciences and Technology, edited by Gary Downey, Joe Dumit, and Sharon Traweek, 83–102. Santa Fe: School of American Research Press.

Dumont, Louis. 1986. *Essays on Individualism.* Chicago: University of Chicago Press.

Emmrich, M. 1994a. "Der schändliche Kannibalismus." *Frankfurter Rundschau,* May 10, p. 7.

———. 1994b. "Der Staat als Organdealer." *Frankfurter Rundschau,* July 28, p. 18.

———. 1994c. "Wenn der Blutdruck der Leiche dramatisch steigt." *Frankfurter Rundschau,* June 27, p. 18.

Eurotransplant Foundation. 1992. *Annual Report.* Leiden.

———. 1993. *Annual Report.* Leiden.

———. 1994. *Newsletter 120.*

Evans, Richard. 1987. *Death in Hamburg.* New York: Cambridge University Press.

Feuerstein, Gunther. 1996. "Body-Recycling Management." In *Körpertechnik: Aufsätze zur Organtransplantation,* edited by Bernward Joerges, 63–138. Berlin: Rainer Bohn Verlag.

Fletcher, Joseph. 1969. "Our Shameful Waste of Human Tissue: An Ethical Problem for the Living and the Dead." In *Updating Life and Death,* edited by Donald Cutler, 1–30. Boston: Beacon.

Flye, M. Wayne, ed. 1995. *Atlas of Organ Transplantation.* Philadelphia: Saunders.

Forsythe, Diana. 1989. "German Identity and Problems of History." In *History and Ethnicity,* edited by Elizabeth Tonkin, Maryon McDonald, and Malcolm Chapman, 137–56. New York: Routledge.

"Fortschritt in der Medizin." 1994. *Bewegte Zeiten.* 112: 16–18.

Foster, Robert. 1991. "Making National Cultures in the Global Ecumene." *Annual Review of Anthropology* 20: 235–60.

Foucault, Michel. 1975. *The Birth of the Clinic: An Archaeology of Medical Perception.* New York: Vintage/Random House.

———. 1979. *Discipline and Punish: The Birth of the Prison.* New York: Vintage/Random House.

Fox, Renée, and Judith Swazey. 1974. *The Courage to Fail: A Social View of Organ Transplants and Dialysis.* Chicago: University of Chicago Press.

———. 1992. *Spare Parts.* New York: Oxford University Press.

Frankfurter Allgemeine Zeitung. 1994a. "Blutwäsche in der Neuen Ländern," August 24, p. 196.

———. 1994b. "Seehofer will das geplante Transplantationsgesetz des Bundes nicht in den Wahlkampf hineinziehen," August 13, p. 12.

———. 1994c. "Organspende: 'Scharping zerschlägt unheimlich viel Porzellan.'" July 31.

Frankfurter Rundschau. 1992. "Gehört zu einem Fötus nicht auch eine lebende Mutter?" October 28, p. 18.

Franklin, Sarah. 1992. "Fetal Fascinations: New Dimensions to the Medical-Scientific Construction of Personhood." In *Off-Centre: Feminism and Cultural Studies,* edited by S. Franklin, C. Lury, and J. Stacey, 190–206. London: HarperCollins.

———. 1995. "Science As Culture, Cultures of Science." *Annual Review of Anthropology* 24: 163–84.

Fritsch-Bournazel, Renata. 1992. *Europe and German Unification.* New York: Berg.

Fritz-Vannahme, Joachim. 1994. "Im Sterben den Lebenden helfen." *Die Zeit,* July 22, p. 30.

Fujimura, Joan. 1987. "Constructing Doable Problems in Cancer Research: Articulating Alignment." *Social Studies of Science* 17: 257–93.

Gast, Wolfgang. 1992. "Fötus beendet Klinik-Experiment." *Tageszeitung,* November 17, p. 2.

Geary, Patrick. 1978. *Furta Sacra: Thefts of Relics in the Central Middle Ages.* Princeton: Princeton University Press.

———. 1986. "Sacred Commodities: The Circulation of Medieval Relics." In *The Social Life of Things,* edited by A. Appadurai, pp. 169–94. New York: Cambridge University Press.

Gervais, Karen. 1986. *Redefining Death.* New Haven: Yale University Press.

Gilman, Sander. 1991. *The Jew's Body.* New York: Routledge.

Graupner, Heidrun. 1994. "Gehört der Leib der Gesellschaft?" *Süddeutsches Zeitung,* July 16, p. 17.

Greinert, Renate, and Gisela Wuttke, eds. 1993. *Organspende: Kritische Ansichten zur Transplantationsmedizin.* Göttingen: Lamuv Taschenbuch.

Gudeman, Stephen. 1992. "Remodeling the House of Economics: Culture and Innovation." *American Ethnologist* 19: 141–55.

Gupta, Akhil, and James Ferguson. 1992. "Beyond 'Culture': Space, Identity and the Politics of Difference." *Cultural Anthropology* 7, no. 1: 6–23.

Habermas, Jürgen. 1988. "Concerning the Public Use of History." *New German Critique* 44: 40–50.

Hacking, Ian. 1992. "The Self-Vindication of the Laboratory Sciences." In *Science As Practice and Culture,* edited by Andrew Pickering, 29–66. Chicago: University of Chicago Press.

Hansmann, Henry. 1989. "The Economics and Ethics of Markets for Human Organs." *Journal of Health Politics, Policy, and Law* 14: 57–86.

Haraway, Donna. 1989. "The Biopolitics of Postmodern Bodies." *Differences* 1, no. 1: 3–45.

———. 1991. *Simians, Cyborgs and Women: The Reinvention of Nature.* New York: Routledge.

Harrington, Anne. 1995. "Unmasking Suffering's Masks: Reflections on Old and New Memories of Nazi Medicine." *Daedalus* 125: 181–206.

Hartouni, Valerie. 1991. "Containing Women: Reproductive Discourse in the 1980's." In *Technoculture,* edited by Constance Penley and Andrew Ross, 27–56. Minneapolis: University of Minnesota Press.

Harwood, Jonathan. 1994. *Styles of Scientific Thought: The German Genetics Community, 1900–1933.* Chicago: University of Chicago Press.

Haupt, W., O. Schober, H. Angstwurm, and K. Kunze. 1993. "Die Feststellung des Todes durch den irreversiblen Ausfall des gesamten Gehirns." *Deutsches Ärzteblatt* 90: B2222–25.

Heath, Deborah. 1998. "Locating Genetic Knowledge: Picturing Marfan Syndrome and Its Travelling Constituencies. *Science, Technology, and Human Values* 23: 71–97.

Helmers, Sabine. 1989. *Tabu und Faszination: Über die Ambivalenz der Einstellung zu Toten.* Berlin: Dietrich Reimer Verlag.

Herf, Jeffrey. 1984. *Reactionary Modernism: Technology, Culture and Politics in Weimar and the Third Reich.* New York: Cambridge University Press.

Hertz, Robert. [1907] 1960. *Death and the Right Hand.* Glencoe, Ill.: Free Press.

Hess, David. 1992. "The New Ethnography and the Anthropology of Science and Technology." In *Knowledge and Society: The Anthropology of Science and Technology,* edited by David Hess and Linda Layne. Greenwich, Conn.: JAI.

———. 1996. *Science and Technology in a Multicultural World.* New York: Columbia University Press.

Hirschauer, Stefan. 1991. "The Manufacture of Bodies in Surgery." *Social Studies of Science* 21: 279–319.

Hobsbawm, Eric J., and Terence Ranger, eds. 1983. *The Invention of Tradition.* Cambridge: Cambridge University Press.

Hoefling, Wolfgang. 1994. "Hinter dem Hirntodkonzept steckt ein reduziertes Menchenbild." *Frankfurter Rundschau,* August 10, p. 16.

Hoff, Johannes, and Jürgen in der Schmitten, eds. 1994. *Wann ist der Mensch Tot?* Hamburg: Rohwolt Verlag.

Hogle, Linda F. 1992. "Body Repairs and Social Reparations." Unpublished manuscript.

———. 1993. "Margins of Life, Boundaries of the Body." Paper presented at a meeting of the Society for Applied Anthropology, San Antonio.

———. 1995a. "Embodied Technologies: Human Materials As Therapeutic and Research Tools." Paper presented at a meeting of the American Anthropological Association, Washington, D.C.

———. 1995b. "Standardization across Non-Standard Domains: The Case of Organ Procurement." *Science, Technology, and Human Values* 20: 482–500.

———. 1995c. "Tales from the Cryptic: Technology Meets Organism in the 'Living Cadaver.'" In *The Cyborg Handbook,* edited by Chris Gray, 203–18. New York: Routledge.

———. 1996. "Die Arbeit am Körper." In *Körpertechnik: Aufsatze zur Organtransplantation,* edited by Bernward Joerges, 185–208. Berlin: Rainer Bohn Verlag.

Huyssen, Andreas. 1995. *Twilight Memories: Marking Time in a Culture of Amnesia.* New York: Routledge.

Iserson, Kenneth. 1994. *Death to Dust: What Happens to Dead Bodies?* Tucson: Galen.

Jaeckel, Gerhard. 1986. *Die Charité.* Frankfurt: Ullstein.

Jasanoff, Sheila. 1995. *Science at the Bar: Law, Science and Technology in America.* Cambridge: Harvard University Press.

Jennett, Brian. 1985. "High-Tech Medicine: How Defined and How Regarded." *Milbank Memorial Fund Quarterly* 63: 141–73.

Jonas, Hans. 1974. *Philosophical Essays: From Ancient Creed to Technological Man.* Englewood Cliffs, N.J.: Prentice Hall.

Joralemon, D. 1995. "Organ Wars: The Battle for Body Parts." *Medical Anthropology Quarterly* 9: 335–56.

Jörns, K. P. 1993. "Organtransplantation, Eine Anfrage an unser Verständnis von Sterben, Tod und Auferstehung." *Berliner Theologische Zeitschrift* 15–39.

Judt, Tony. 1992. "The Past Is Another Country: Myth and Memory in Postwar Europe." *Daedalus* 121: 83–118.

Kaes, Anton. 1989. *From Hitler to Heimat.* Cambridge: Harvard University Press.

Kahn, Patricia. 1992. "Germany's Gene Law Begins to Bite." *Science* 255: 524–26.

———. 1995. "Blending Biology, Technology and Economic Development." *Science* 267: 785.

Kater, M. 1987. "The Burden of the Past: Problems of a Modern Historiography of Physicians and Medicine in Nazi Germany." *German Studies Review* 10: 31–56.

Kaufman, H. 1986. "Brain Death." *Neurosurgery* 19: 850–56.

Kimbrell, Andrew. 1993. *The Human Body Shop: The Engineering and Marketing of Life.* San Francisco: Harper.

Klein, Martin. 1995. "Hirntod: Vollständiger und irreversibler Verlust aller Hirnfunktionen?" *Ethik in der Medizin* 7: 6–15.

Klinkmueller, Erich. 1986. "The Medical Industrial Complex." In *Political Values and Health Care: The German Experience,* edited by Donald Light and Alexander Schuller, 53–72. Cambridge: MIT Press.

Knorr-Cetina, Karin. 1981. *The Manufacture of Knowledge: An Essay on the Constructivist and Contextual Nature of Science.* New York: Pergamon.

Koebe, H. G., and F. W. Schildberg. 1994. "Cell Supply for Hybrid Liver Assist Devices." Paper presented at the Symposium for New Transplantation Technology, Bad Oeynhausen, Germany, September 6–8.

Koenig, Barbara. 1988. "The Technological Imperative in Medical Practice: The Social Creation of a 'Routine' Treatment." In *Biomedicine Examined,* edited by Margaret Lock and Deborah Gordon, 465–96. London: Kluwer.

Kohler, Robert E. 1994. *Lords of the Fly: Drosophila Genetics and the Experimental Life.* Chicago: University of Chicago Press.

Kommers, Donald. 1995. "Building Democracy: Judicial Review and the German Rechstaat." Paper presented at the Center for German and Western European Studies Symposium, University of California, Berkeley, November.

Kopytoff, Igor. 1986. "The Cultural Biography of Things: Commoditization As Process." In *The Social Life of Things,* edited by Arjun Appadurai, 64–94. New York: Cambridge University Press.

Korb, S., G. Albornoz, W. Brems, A. Ali, and J. A. Light. 1989. "Verapamil Pretreatment of Hemodynamically Unstable Donors Prevents Delayed Graft Function Post-Transplant." *Transplantation Proceedings* 21: 1236–38.

Kramer, Jane. 1996. *The Politics of Memory.* New York: Random House.

Kruska, Wolfgang. 1994. "Trotzdem müssen wir miteinander auskommen!" *Berliner Ärzte* 10: 11–22.

Kuratorium für Hemodialyse. 1993. *Jahresbericht.* Frankfurt.

Lamb, David. 1985. *Death, Brain Death and Ethics.* Albany: SUNY Press.

Land, Walter, and Bernard Cohen. 1992. "Postmortem and Living Organ Donation in Europe: Transplant Laws and Activities." *Transplantation Proceedings* 24, no. 5: 2165–67.

Langbein, Hermann. 1972. *Menschen in Auschwitz*. Vienna: Europaverlag.

Laqueur, Thomas. 1983. "Bodies, Death and Pauper Funerals." *Representations* 1: 109–30.

Latour, Bruno. 1987. *Science in Action: How to Follow Scientists and Engineers Through Society*. Cambridge: Harvard University Press.

Latour, Bruno, and Steve Woolgar. 1979. *Laboratory Life: The Social Construction of Scientific Facts*. Beverly Hills, Calif.: Sage.

Lenoir, Timothy. 1997. *Instituting Science: The Cultural Production of Scientific Disciplines*. Stanford: Stanford University Press.

Lifton, Robert Jay. 1986. *The Nazi Doctors*. New York: Basic Books.

Linke, Ulrike. 1986. "Where Blood Flows, a Tree Grows: A Study of Root Metaphors in German Culture." Ph.D. diss., University of California.

———. 1995a. "Formations of White Public Space: German Citizenship Laws, Refugee Politics and the Bodily Imaginary." Paper presented at a meeting of the American Anthropological Association, Washington D.C., November 15–19.

———. 1995b. "Murderous Fantasies: Violence, Memory and Selfhood in Germany." *New German Critique* 64: 37–60.

Lock, Margaret. 1993. *Encounters with Aging: Mythologies of Menopause in Japan and North America*. Berkeley: University of California Press.

———. 1995. "Contesting the Natural in Japan: Moral Dilemmas and Technologies of the Dying." *Culture, Medicine, and Psychiatry* 19: 1–38.

———. 1996. "Deadly Disputes: Ideologies and Brain Death in Japan." In *Organ Transplantation: Meanings and Realities*, edited by Stuart Youngner, Renée Fox, and Laurence O'Connell, 142–67. Madison: University of Wisconsin Press.

Lock, Margaret, and Christine Honde. 1990. "Reaching Consensus about Death: Heart Transplants and Cultural Identity in Japan." In *Social Science Perspectives on Medical Ethics*, edited by George Weisz, 99–120. Philadelphia: University of Pennsylvania Press.

Lynch, Michael. 1985. *Art and Artifact in Laboratory Science: A Study of Shop Work and Shop Talk in a Research Laboratory*. London: Routledge and Kegan Paul.

———. 1988. "Sacrifice and the Transformation of the Animal Body into a Scientific Object." *Social Studies of Science* 18: 265–89.

McKenzie, Nancy. 1990. "Oil and Water? A United German Health Care System." *Health/PAC Bulletin* (Winter): 21–23.

McLain, Linda. 1995. "Inviolability and Privacy: The Castle, the Sanctuary and the Body." *Yale Journal of Law and the Humanities* 7: 195–241.

Maier, Charles. 1988. *The Unmasterable Past: History, Holocaust and German National Identity*. Cambridge: Harvard University Press.

Marcus, George. 1986. "Contemporary Problems of Ethnography in the Modern World System." In *Writing Culture*, edited by J. Clifford and G. Marcus, 165–93. Berkeley: University of California Press.

Marcus, George, and Michael Fischer. 1986. *Anthropology As Cultural Critique*. Chicago: University of Chicago Press.

Markovits, Andrei. 1988. "Introduction to the Broszat/Friedländer Exchange." *New German Critique* 44: 81–84.

Marshall, Patricia, David Thomasma, and Abdullah Daar. 1996. "Marketing Human Organs: The Autonomy Paradox." *Theoretical Medicine* 17: 1–18.

Martin, Emily. 1992. "The End of the Body?" *American Ethnologist* 19: 121–40.

——. 1994. *Flexible Bodies*. Boston: Beacon.

——. 1998. "Anthropology and the Cultural Study of Science." *Science, Technology, and Human Values* 23: 24–44.

Mathieu, Deborah, ed. 1988. *Organ Substitution Technology: Ethical, Legal and Public Policy Issues*. Boulder, Colo.: Westview.

Matschke, K., S. M. Tugtekin, F. Wagner, H. R. Zerkowski, F. Mohr, and S. Schuler. 1997. "A New Form of Donor Allocation: Mid-German Transplant Units." *Transplantation Proceedings* 29: 3430.

Meran, J., and S. Poliwada. 1992. "Der Hirntod und das Ende menschlichen Lebens." *Ethik in der Medizin* 4: 165–71.

——. 1994. "Leben und sterben lassen: Anthropologie und Pragmatik des Hirntodes." In *Wann ist der Mensch Tot?*, edited by J. Hoff and J. in der Schmitten, 68–81. Hamburg: Rowohlt.

Metcalf, Peter, and Richard Huntington. 1991. *Celebrations of Death: The Anthropology of Mortuary Ritual*. 2d ed. New York: Cambridge University Press.

Mitford, Jessica. 1963. *The American Way of Death*. New York: Simon and Schuster.

Mitscherlich, Alexander. 1949. *Doctors of Infamy: The Story of the Nazi Medical Crimes*. New York: Schuman.

Mosse, George. [1964] 1981. *The Crisis of German Ideology*. New York: Schocken.

Motoyama, K., T. Kamei, Y. Nakafusa, M. Ueki, et al. 1995. "Donor Treatment with Gadolinium Chloride Improves Survival after Transplantation of Cold-Stored Livers by Reducing Kupffer Cell Tumor Necrosis Factor Production in Rats." *Transplantation Proceedings* 27: 762–64.

Mueller-Hill, Benno. 1988. *Murderous Science*. New York: Oxford University Press.

Murphy, Julian. 1989. "Should Pregnancies Be Allowed in Brain-Dead Women? A Philosophical Discussion of Postmortem Pregnancy." In *Healing Technology*, edited by Katherine Ratcliff, 135–59. Ann Arbor: University of Michigan Press.

Neiburg, F., and M. Goldman. 1998. "Anthropology and Politics in Studies of National Character." *Cultural Anthropology* 13: 56–81.

New York Times. 1991. "Video Game Uncovered in Europe Uses Nazi Death Camps As Theme," May 1, p. A10.

——. 1994. "Five Years Later: Germany Remains Sharply Divided and Resentment Festers." October 14, p. A1.

Novitzky, D., K. C. Cooper, and B. Reichart. 1987. "Hemodynamic and Metabolic Responses to Hormonal Therapy in Brain-Dead Potential Organ Donors." *Transplantation* 43: 852–54.

Novitzky, D., K. C. Cooper, A. G. Rose, and B. Reichart. 1987. "Prevention of Myocardial Injury by Pretreatment with Verapamil Hydrochloride Prior to Experimental Brain Death: Efficacy in a Baboon Model." *American Journal of Emergency Medicine* 5: 11–18.

Ohnuki-Tierney, Emiko. 1994. "Brain Death and Organ Transplantation: Cultural Bases of Medical Technology." *Current Anthropology* 35: 233–54.

Opelz, G. 1992. "The Collaborative Transplant Study: Ten Year Report." *Transplantation Proceedings* 24: 2342–55.

Parham, P. 1993. "HLA, Anthropology and Transplantation." *Transplantation Proceedings* 25, no. 1: 159–61.

Park, Katherine. 1994. "The Criminal and the Saintly Body." *Renaissance Quarterly* 47: 1–33.

———. 1995. "The Life of the Corpse: Division and Dissection in Late Medieval Europe." *Journal of the History of Medicine* 50: 111–32.

Pernick, Martin. 1988. "Back from the Grave: Recurring Controversies over Defining and Diagnosing Death in History." In *Death: Beyond Whole Brain Criteria*, edited by Richard Zaner, 17–74. Boston: Kluwer.

Peters, Hermann. 1924. *Der Arzt und die Heilkraft in der deutschen Vergangenheit.* Jena: Eugen Diederichs Verlag.

Pichlmayr, R. 1991. *Lebenschance Organtransplantation: Wissenswertes über Durchführung und Probleme von Organtransplantationen.* Stuttgart: Thieme.

Pickering, Andrew, ed. 1992. *Science As Practice and Culture.* Chicago: University of Chicago Press.

Pine, V. R. 1975. *Caretaker of the Dead.* New York: Irvington.

Plough, Alonzo. 1981. "Medical Technology and the Crisis of Experience: The Costs of Clinical Legitimation." *Social Science and Medicine* 15F: 89–101.

———. 1986. *Borrowed Time: Artificial Organs and the Politics of Extending Lives.* Philadelphia: Temple University Press.

Poster, Mark. 1990. *The Mode of Information: Poststructuralism and Social Context.* Chicago: University of Chicago Press.

Proctor, Robert. 1988. *Racial Hygiene: Medicine under the Nazis.* Cambridge: Harvard University Press.

Pross, Christian, and Goetz Aly. 1989. *Der Wert des Menschen: Medizin in Deutschland, 1918–1945.* Berlin: Hentrich.

Prottas, R. 1985. "Organ Procurement in Europe and the U.S." *Milbank Memorial Quarterly* 63, no. 1: 94–126.

Rabinow, Paul. 1992a. "Artificiality and Enlightenment: from Sociobiology to Biosociality." In *Incorporations: Zone 6*, edited by J. Crary and S. Kwinter. New York: Urzone.

———. 1992b. "Severing the Ties: Fragmentation and Dignity in Late Modernity." *Knowledge and Society: The Anthropology of Science and Technology* 9: 169–87.

Radin, Margaret Jane. 1996. *Contested Commodities.* Cambridge: Harvard University Press.

Ranke-Heinemann, Ute. 1992. "Menschenwürde, ein Totschlage Wort." *Tageszeitung*, October 23, p. 10.

Rapp, Rayna. 1988. "Chromosomes and Communication: The Discourse of Genetic Counselling." *Medical Anthropology Quarterly* 2: 143–57.

Reiser, Stanley. 1978. *Medicine and the Reign of Technology.* Cambridge: Cambridge University Press.

Rettig, Richard. 1989. "The Politics of Organ Transplantation: A Parable for Our Time." *Journal of Health Politics, Policy, and Law* 14: 191–221.

Rheinz, Hanna. 1992. "Der Mensch als Recyclingobjekt." *Wochenpost* 53: 28–29.

Richardson, Ruth. 1989. *Death, Dissection and the Destitute.* New York: Routledge.

Ropper, A. H. 1984. "Unusual Spontaneous Movements." *Neurology* 34: 1089.

Rothman, David. 1991. *Strangers at the Bedside.* New York: Basic Books.

Rupp, Jan. 1992. "Michel Foucault, Body Politics and the Rise and Expansion of Modern Anatomy." *Journal of Historical Sociology* 5, no. 1: 31–59.

San Francisco Chronicle. 1993. "Germans to Defend Corpse Crash Tests," November 25, p. 18.

Schaefer, Dietrich. 1920. "Mittelalterlicher Brauch bei der Überführung von Leichen." In *Sitzungsberichte der preussischer Akademie der Wissenschaft,* 478–98. Frankfurt: Suhrkamp.

Scheper-Hughes, Nancy. 1996. "Theft of Life: The Globalization of Organ Stealing Rumors." *Anthropology Today* 12: 3–11.

Scheper-Hughes, Nancy, and Margaret Lock. 1987. "The Mindful Body: A Prolegomenon to Future Work in Medical Anthropology." *Medical Anthropology Quarterly* 1: 6–41.

Schildhauer, Johannes. 1988. *The Hansa.* Leipzig: Dorset.

Schlaes, Amity. 1995. "A Germany That Kills Science." *Wall Street Journal,* November 7.

Schmidt, Helmut. 1994. "Anzahl der Dialyse-Zentren hat sich in den neuen Bundesländern verdoppelt." *Berliner Ärzteblatt* 107: 445–46.

Schmidt, Volker. 1996. *Politik der Organverteilung: Eine Untersuchung Über Empfängerauswahl in der Transplantationsmedizin.* Baden-Baden: Nomos.

———. 1998. "Selection of Recipients for Donor Organs in Transplant Medicine." *Journal of Medicine and Philosophy* 23: 50–74.

Schmidt, Walter. 1993. "The Nation in German History." In *The National Question in Europe in Historical Context,* edited by Mikulás Teich and Roy Porter. New York: Cambridge University Press.

Schütt, G., H. Smit, and P. Schroeder. 1992. "Organizational Structures As the Basis for Successful Kidney Transplantation in Germany." *Transplantation Proceedings* 24, no. 5: 2052–53.

Schütt, G., H. Smit, and G. Duncker. 1995. "Huge Discrepancy between Declared Support of Organ Donation and Actual Rate of Consent for Organ Retrieval." *Transplantation Proceedings* 27, no. 1: 1450–51.

Scott, Russell. 1981. *The Body As Property.* New York: Viking.

Shapin, Steven. 1994. *A Social History of Truth.* Chicago: University of Chicago Press.

Sharp, Lesley. 1995. "Organ Transplantation As Transformative Experience: Anthropological Insights into the Restructuring of the Self." *Medical Anthropology Quarterly* 9: 357–89.

———. 1998. "Remembering and Memorializing the Dead after Organ Donation." Paper presented at the annual meeting of the American Anthropological Association, Philadelphia, December.

Singer, Peter. 1994. *Rethinking Life and Death: The Collapse of Our Traditional Ethics.* New York: St. Martin's.

Soifer, B., and A. Gelb. 1989. "The Multiple Organ Donor: Identification and Management." *Annals of Internal Medicine* 110: 814–23.

Stein, Rosemarie. 1992. *Die Charité, 1945–1992.* Berlin: Argon Verlag.

Stone, Allucquere Rosanne. 1992. "Will the Real Body Please Stand Up? Boundary Stories about Virtual Culture." In *Cyberspace: First Steps,* edited by M. Benedikt, 81–118. Cambridge: MIT Press.

Stone, Deborah. 1991. "German Unification: East Meets West in the Doctor's Office." *Journal of Health Politics, Policy, and Law* 16, no. 2: 401–11.

Strack, Hermann. 1909. *The Jew and Human Sacrifice in History: Sociological Inquiry.* New York: Bloch.

Strathern, Marilyn. 1992. *Reproducing the Future: Anthropology, Kinship and the New Reproductive Technologies.* New York: Routledge.

Strauss, Anselm, Shizuko Fagerhaugh, Barbara Suczek, and Carolyn Wiener. 1985. *The Social Organization of Medical Work.* Chicago: University of Chicago Press.

Striebel, Hans-Walter, and Jurgen Link, eds. 1993. *Ich Pflege Tote: Die Andere Seite der Transplantationsmedizin.* Basel: Recom Verlag.

Tagespiegel. 1992. "Erlanger Baby nach natürlichen Abort tot," November 17, p. 30.

Tageszeitung. 1992. "Abgang des Erlanger Fötus; tote Mutter abgeschaltet," November 17, pp. 1–2.

Tambiah, Stanley. 1990. *Magic, Science and Religion.* Cambridge: Cambridge University Press.

Taupitz, Joachim. 1994. "Zum Umgang mit der Leiche in der Medizin." *Ethik in der Medizin* 6: 38–42.

Thaw, H. 1994. "Reperfusion Damage in Donor Organs." In *Organ Preservation: Basic and Applied Aspects,* edited by D. E. Pegg, I. A. Jacobson, and N. A. Halasy. Philadelphia: Saunders.

Thomas, Hans. 1993. "Ehrfürcht vor dem Leib oder Fürcht vor der Medizin." *Medizinische Klinik* 88: 39–44.

Thompson, John. 1995. "American Society of Histocompatibility and Immunogenetics Crossmatch Study." *New England Journal of Medicine* 59, no. 11: 1636–37.

Turner, Bryan. 1987. *The Body and Society.* Oxford: Blackwell.

———. 1992. *Regulating Bodies.* New York: Q≤utledge.

Ulrich, B., and F. Geschonneck. 1994. "Stört Organentnahme die Totenruhe?" *Berliner Zeitung,* February 24, p. 5.

United Network for Organ Sharing. 1994. *UNOS Bulletin* 10: 14.

Van Gennep, Arnold. [1909] 1960. *The Rites of Passage.* Chicago: University of Chicago Press.

Veatch, Robert. 1988. *Death, Dying and the Biological Revolution.* New Haven: Yale University Press.

Vollmer, Rainer. 1994. "Ärtze müssen mit einem neuen europaeischen Haftungsrecht rechnen." *Ärzte Zeitung,* August 29, p. 151.

Wechsler, Andrew. 1989. "Free Radicals: The Reperfusion Ninja." *Annals of Thoracic Surgery* 47: 798.

Weindling, Paul. 1989. *Health, Race and German Politics between National Unification and Nazism, 1870–1945.* New York: Cambridge University Press.

Weingart, Peter, Jürgen Kroll, and Kurt Bayertz. 1988. *Rasse, Blut und Gene: Geschichte der Eugenik und Rassenhygiene in Deutschland.* Frankfurt: Suhrkamp.

Wetzel, R., N. Setzer, J. Stiff, and M. Rogers. 1985. "Hemodynamic Responses in Brain Dead Organ Donor Patients." *Anesthesia and Analgesia* 64: 125–28.

Wiesemann, C. 1995. "Hirntod und Gesellschaft." *Ethik in der Medizin* 7: 16–28.

Wijnen, R.M.H., and C. J. van der Linden. 1991. "Donor Treatment after Pronouncement of Brain Death: A Neglected Intensive Care Problem." *Transplant International* 4: 186–90.

Wuermeling, Hans-Bernhard. 1992. "Das Kind in der toten Mutter." *Frankfurter Allgemeine Zeitung,* October 17, p. 9.

Wuttke, Gisela. 1991. "Spenderorgane: Schäppchen für die Chirurgie." *Tagezeitung,* September 9, p. 19.

Youngner, Stuart. 1990. "Organ Retrieval: Can We Ignore the Dark Side?" *Transplantation Proceedings* 22, no. 3: 1014–15.

Youngner, Stuart, Renée Fox, and Laurence O'Connell, eds. 1996. *Organ Transplantation: Meanings and Reality.* Madison: University of Wisconsin Press.

Index

abortion, 62, 64, 207*n*4, 208*n*1
allocation systems, 76, 105, 113;
  center-driven, 131; manipulation
  of, 131, 132, 133; patient-driven,
  131; by perfect match, 130;
  regional priorities in, 130–131;
  rotational, 130, 131; by sickest
  patient, 130–131; time priorities in,
  131–132
altruism, 2, 43, 76, 77, 191, 195,
  208*n*14
Angstwurm, H., 82
animation, 24, 28–33, 40, 60, 165;
  constructed definitions of, 63–67;
  continued, 3, 24, 41, 80, 190
Appadurai, Arjun, 15
Aquinas, Thomas, 29
Arbeitsgemeinschaft der Deutschen
  Transplantation Zentren e.V., 112
Arbeitskreis Organspende, 112
Ariès, Philippe, 28, 32, 38, 39
Arzneimittel (pharmaceuticals), 109,
  119
Austria, 11, 69*tab*, 104, 144
autonomy, 14, 23, 90
autopsy: laws, 69, 74, 87; tissue
  procurement at, 134

Bahrrecht, 32
Basic Law (West Germany, 1949), 55,
  58, 60–63, 78, 79, 188, 189
Battaglia, Debbora, 25, 26
Baudrillard, Jean, 189, 190
Bauman, Zygmunt, 189, 195
Beleidigung (insult to the dead), 157
Belgium, 11, 69*tab*, 104
Berg, Marc, 140, 214*n*14
Berliner Initiative, 89
Bierrecht, 32
Binski, Paul, 34
bioethics, 193–194, 206*n*7
BioImplant Services, 108, 109, 136,
  198, 210*n*11, 217
Birnbacher, D., 82
Bloch, Maurice, 25
blood, 38–39; *Blut und Boden* slogan,
  48; cults, 204*n*3; as symbol, 48
Blut und Boden, 48
body: accessibility, 42; animation, 24,
  28–33, 40; boundaries of, 6;
  collectible, 3, 35–38, 51–53;
  commemoration of, 27, 28, 190,
  191, 204*n*4; as commodity, 6, 8, 23,
  24, 42; conceptions of, 19–20,
  201*n*3; continued animation in, 3,

233

58, 190, 195–196; medical abuses
under, 1, 73, 159; medical membership, 206n8; social-medical
projects of, 3, 45–58 *passim*
Neiberg, F., 9

Ohnuki-Tierney, Emiko, 7, 207n7
Opelz, G., 103, 132
Organhandel (organ sales), 88
Organizationzentrale (coordinating
organization), 97
organ procurement/donation: as act
of commemoration, 27, 28, 190,
191, 204n4; automatic, 89; center-
driven, 99, 131; centralization of,
85, 103; clinical measurements
during, 147–151; commercialization of, 7, 23, 24, 33, 91, 109;
contraindications for, 146; costs of,
7, 114, 211n14; cultural practices
and, 180–185; decrease in, 15;
diversity of practices, 130; donor
eligibility, 142–144; as duty/
obligation, 77, 89, 90, 189, 191–
192; ethical considerations, 7; in
Europe, 104–107; evaluating
sources, 43; from foreigners, 144;
German views on, 11; in Germany,
106–107, 111–122, 153–160, 197–
199; historical background, 116–
119; infectious agents and, 31, 39,
87, 143; infrastructure of, 7, 102–
111; international rates, 106–107;
local practice, 124–139; medical
practices and, 180–185; negative
perceptions of, 91, 112, 126, 127,
135; organization of, 73, 99–123,
101–123, 161; patient-driven, 99;
procedures, 4, 161–185; protocols,
161; public promotion of, 112, 136;
regional/local variations in, 96,
115, 116–119; regional organizations, 97, 99; removal procedures,
96, 97, 174–180; reporting
potential donors, 126–127; rotation

system for allocation, 130, 131;
sources of, 98, 101–102, 142–144;
technical constraints of, 7;
transnational infrastructure, 102–
111; in transplant centers, 124–
125; transport issues, 98; in United
States, 43, 126, 142–152, 197–199;
vulnerable populations and, 5. *See
also* Deutsche Stiftung für
Organspende; donor management;
Eurotransplant
organs: accept/reject decisions, 103,
129, 133, 168–174, 176; aggressive
attempts to procure, 5, 7; allocation of, 20, 76, 105, 113, 130;
control over, 122; demand for, 4, 5,
87, 111; differing beliefs about, 10;
experiments on, 49–51, 83, 85;
failure of, 4; matching (*see* tissue
matching); preservation techniques, 95, 102, 132, 149–152,
214n13; "prime-quality," 151;
protection therapy, 157–158;
reserve capacity in, 171; sale of,
86–88, 195; sharing, 131; shortage
of, 77, 111. *See also* human
biological materials

Park, Katherine, 30, 34, 36, 38
Parry, Jonathan, 25
Pernick, Martin, 32, 33
personhood, 41, 68; disturbance of,
90; formulation of, 76; laws, 55, 60–
61, 75, 81; protection of, 60–63; of
removed body parts, 7, 24, 40–41,
83–84; rights of, 73
Persönlichkeitsrechte (personhood
laws), 60–63
Pietätsempfinden (reverence for the
dead), 61, 75, 81, 218
Ploch, Marian, 80–83
Poland, 111, 210n6
policy: biological approaches to, 47;
population, 47; pronatal, 48; racial,
47, 48, 210n3, 213n4;

Spain, 69*tab,* 198*tab,* 210*n*7
standardization: European Union and,
10, 109–110; of policies, 10, 174; of
procedures, 9, 109–110, 151, 174
Störung der Totenruhe (disturbing the
dead), 35, 61, 75, 86, 159, 218
Strack, Hermann, 39
Strafgesetz (penal code), 61
Strathern, Marilyn, 6, 152
Striebel, Hans-Walter, 66, 83
Swazey, Judith, 7

Tambiah, Stanley, 36
Taupitz, Joachim, 83
technology, 192–194; alteration of
death process and, 26, 80–83;
appropriate application of, 80;
artificial support, 60, 67, 80–83, 96,
127; cellular, 204*n*2; commercialization of, 7, 91; communication,
180; contested, 91, 92; effect on
society, 5; enhancement, 152;
evaluative, 173; gene, 202*n*16;
imaging, 148; immunosuppressive,
132; impact on the body, 140; as
industrial mainstay, 11–12;
material body and, 68; relation to
body, 5; resuscitative, 26, 32, 33,
64, 65, 213*n*9
Thomas, Hans, 67
tissue banks, 108–110, 119
tissue matching, 95, 99, 102–103, 113,
127, 130, 132, 210*n*3. *See also*
human leukocytic antigens
tissue procurement, 134–139; at
autopsy, 135; bone, 135, 137, 178,
198; cornea, 135, 137, 178, 198; in
Europe, 107–110; in Germany,
119–122; infectious agents and, 31,
39, 87, 109, 143, 206*n*4; laws on,
69; quality/safety standards, 108–
110, 151; regulation of, 68, 109;
skin, 135, 137, 138, 178, 198;
surgical, 135, 138
tissues: accept/reject decisions, 103,

129, 133, 168–174, 176; allocation
of, 76, 113, 130; cadaver, 74–76;
culture medium, 51; demand for, 4,
5, 87; differing beliefs about, 10;
donor registries, 108; exchange of,
107–110, 119–120; grafting, 50;
preservation of, 95, 102, 132, 149–
152; regeneration of, 50; removal
of, for research, 120, 121; sale of,
86–88, 195; shortage of, 77, 111;
storage/banking of, 95, 108–110,
119–120, 122, 138; substitution, 4.
See also human biological materials
Toten (the dead), 63
Totensontag (Memorial Day), 27
Totensorgerecht (right to care for the
dead), 35, 218
transmigration, 29
transplantation: centers, 73, 97, 98,
99, 103, 104–105, 111, 124, 130,
131; clinical management, 96–99,
149–160; continued animation and,
190; costs of, 7, 114, 211*n*14,
212*n*94; laws on, 67–74; profitability of, 12, 133; redemption in, 30,
43; regulation of, 68, 73; social
science perspectives, 7; as
technological solution, 4; waiting
lists, 98, 103, 105, 131
Transplantation Koordinatoren. See
coordinators
Transplantationskodex, 211*n*21
transport issues, 98, 103, 168, 181,
210*n*5
Turner, Bryan, 5, 201*n*1, 205*nn*7, 8,
207*n*5

Übermensch, 90
Ulrich, B., 88
Uniform Determination of Death Act
(U.S., 1981), 65
United Network for Organ Sharing
(U.S.), 97, 98, 145, 179, 212*n*4, 218
United States: accept/reject deci-
sions, 168, 172; burial practices,

About the Author

Linda F. Hogle is an anthropologist who writes and teaches about the anthropology of science, technology, and medicine as well as bioethics and cultural diversity. In addition to two ethnographic studies of organ and tissue procurement, she has researched legal, cultural, and ethical issues in emerging cell and gene technologies. She is a fellow at the Stanford University Center for Biomedical Ethics.